RAW
FOOD
made simple

KAREN KNOWLER

RAW FOOD MADE SIMPLE

First published in the United Kingdom in 2010 by Raw Food Coach Media.
Copyright © Karen Knowler 2010. All rights reserved.

Karen Knowler has asserted her right under the Copyright, Designs and
Patent Act 1988 to be identified as the author of this work.

ISBN 978-0-9567256-0-8

Concept design, layout and print by Pentacor plc, High Wycombe
www.pentacorbookdesign.co.uk

Disclaimer
The techniques and advice described in this book represent the opinions
of the author based on her experience. The author and publisher
expressly disclaim any responsibility for any liability, loss or risk, personal
or otherwise, which is incurred as a result of using any of the techniques,
recipes or recommendations suggested herein. If in any doubt, or if
requiring medical advice, please contact the appropriate health care
professional.

Contents

Introduction   3

chapter 1   So what is raw food and "The Raw Food Diet"?   7

chapter 2   Benefits, benefits   11

chapter 3   All or nothing?   17

chapter 4   "So what do you eat?"   23

chapter 5   Making the change   31

chapter 6   Equipping your kitchen   43

chapter 7   Raw shopping   49

chapter 8   Raw food nutrition   59

chapter 9   Family & social situations   71

chapter 10   Time, money & energy issues   83

chapter 11   Your 5 day raw lifestyle plan   93

chapter 12   Go raw! action steps summary   117

chapter 13   Final word: it's your story – you decide   125

chapter 14   15 quick, easy & delicious raw food recipes   129

chapter 15   Raw transformation stories   151

About the author   175
Want more raw?   177
If you love this book…   178
Wholesale enquiries   179
Thank you   181

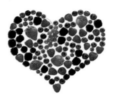

To lovers of life everywhere.

Introduction

"Raw food", "the raw food diet", "going raw" – perhaps you've heard these terms already or maybe you've only just come across them, but what exactly do they mean?

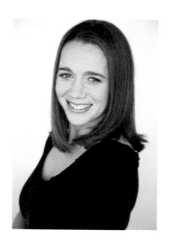

You're here because you're either new to raw food and don't yet know what it's all about, or you're already raw food savvy and are checking to see if you have the basics down. Either way, kudos to you. It takes a certain type of person to be open enough to entertain something that is still seen by many as unusual, "extreme", trendy or faddy (and they're the polite terms!).

Welcome! My name is Karen Knowler, also known as "The Raw Food Coach", and it is my honour and pleasure to be your guide on the short but comprehensive trip we are about to take around the fascinating topic of raw food.

If you've been confused as to what raw food is all about or even if this is the first time you've heard about it, don't worry, you're certainly not alone. Like most topics there's a whole world of information out there about raw food and "the raw food diet", but it's knowing which bits are useful to you and which bits you can trust that's important. I'm here to give you all of that, quickly, easily and in a way that makes total sense so you can see if eating more raw food is for you. If you're anything like I was when I got started, then you may be surprised at just how easy raw food really is and how much sense it makes when you see what it's all about.

If my name is new to you, then feel free to check me out at **www.TheRawFoodCoach.com**. There you can read my story (my background may well surprise you!) and how I went from being a raw food rookie to being a fully-fledged international raw food coach, chef and trainer – it's amazing what can happen when you get passionate about something. I'm here to share with you just why raw food gets people passionate, which, I'm more than well aware, can be hard to imagine when most people think it's all about carrots and apples...

In this book I'll be addressing the carrots and apples and all of those early questions that you're likely to be asking – in fact you'll probably think that I'm reading your mind!

By the end of the book not only will you have a complete and accurate picture of what raw food is and isn't, but you'll also be in a position to give it a whirl – a little or a lot – if it sounds like something you want to explore for yourself.

It's time to make raw food deliciously simple.

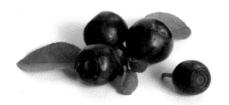

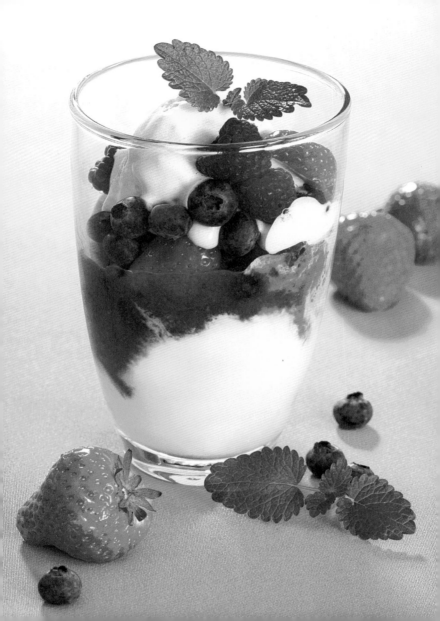

chapter 1
So what is raw food and "The Raw Food Diet"?

Raw food is, generally speaking, food that has not been heated above 48 degrees centigrade (117 degrees Fahrenheit). This usually means uncooked foods, or, more specifically, foods in their natural state – nothing more, nothing less.

By default this will mean foods that are safe to eat raw, which are the obvious foods like fruits, vegetables, nuts and seeds – but there is a whole array of raw foods both within these particular food groups and also many more outside of them that could very well be new to you. We'll be talking about these when we get to the specifics of what to eat in Chapter 4.

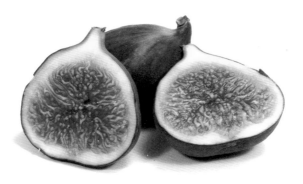

"Raw food", while not being the most attractive term perhaps, is, at least for now, the most accurate. You may also have heard the term "living" or "live" food – this is often used interchangeably with "raw" in conversation or in writing, usually because it sounds much more appealing (and gives a better idea as to the feeling of eating this way), but technically the term should really only be applied to those foods that are still alive and growing, like sprouted beans and seeds, and the foods which are commonly referred to as "indoor greens", such as wheatgrass, sunflower greens and pea greens.

What makes raw food so special is that because it hasn't been cooked, it still has all of its nutrients intact and that makes every bite a powerhouse of nutrition and life-force. It goes without saying that a truly "whole" food is going to be better for you than anything else, but there are many more reasons why raw food is so fabulous. We'll be looking at those in more detail in Chapter 8.

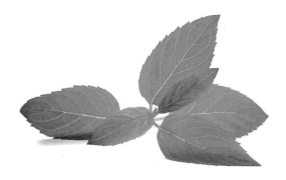

One final myth to bust before we get started: the idea of there being such a thing as "the raw food diet" is actually a huge misnomer, that is unless you think the term "the cooked food diet" is useful or descriptive, because there really are infinite ways to eat raw just as there are infinite ways to eat cooked. Everybody's diet will be different for different reasons and that fine! It's really important to know that. Many people go looking for "the raw food diet" like a Holy Grail that's waiting to be discovered but they never find it – *this is why!* Your diet, just like mine, is whatever you choose to make it – cooked or raw, or a mixture of the two. Your perfect way *will* reveal itself; it's just a case of knowing more about the raw part...

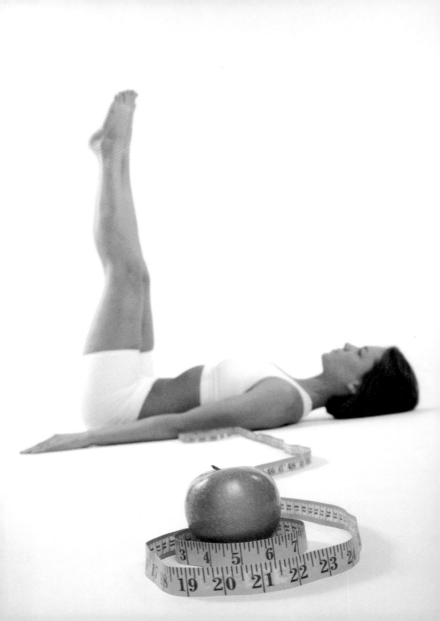

chapter 2
Benefits, benefits

So why do so many people rave about the benefits of raw food? I mean, sure, it must be good for us because of its very nature (fresh, ripe, whole, pure, all of the nutrients still intact and not destroyed or reduced through cooking), but what does this translate to exactly?

I'm glad you asked!

What people tend to find first is that the physical benefits reveal themselves VERY quickly. Granted, this is when people give raw food a "serious" shot, as in, they don't eat burgers and fries all day, add in some lettuce and tomato and then say "there's my raw food – so why don't I feel any better?" You have to give it a chance!

Having said that, it is perfectly reasonable and realistic to expect to see and feel noticeable changes physically in as little as 24 hours.

These changes can be as simple as niggling aches and pains disappearing, through to seeing a difference in body tone, clearer eyes, a less puffy face on waking and all manner of other things. As you might expect, the longer you do it, the more significant the changes. The body just loves to have a good run of it!

It's perhaps not surprising then that those who have been eating mostly raw food or all raw food for a year or more can often look ten years younger than they actually are, be completely rid of those aches and pains and niggling health issues, have shiny hair, glowing skin and sparkling eyes, not to mention a body that looks and functions like something most of us thought we could only ever dream about.

The fact is that we *rejuvenate* on raw and living foods. In the process of replacing our cells and bloodstream with cleaner, better nourished, more "alive" cells, we cannot help but to grow younger and look better. It's pretty straightforward when you think about it. What you put in you *do* get out.

In fact, there are many real life case studies of people who have not only got younger-looking and healthier on raw food, but who have recovered from serious illnesses and disease – in some cases they were only days away from death. Such is the power of raw and living foods when used as medicine as well as food.

> *"Let food be thy medicine and medicine be thy food."*
> Hippocrates

Now, honestly that's just a tiny overview of the physical benefits. Seeing truly is believing, and that's where the fun begins because we can't argue with our own experience. Where it gets even more interesting, however, is in the fact that the benefits of eating raw extend to the emotional, mental and even spiritual for some people.

Allow me to explain...

As you can hopefully appreciate from what I've shared above, as you bring more raw (fresh/alive) foods into your body, the happier and healthier your body gets. Designed for health, radiance and helping you reach your potential as a human being, the body's biggest desire is to embody these things for REAL rather than just hold the capacity for them. It's up to you (the you that drives the vehicle) to decide if you're interested in that – your food choices will either support or deny that reality. It's that simple.

Where it gets fun is that pretty soon after starting to eat more raw you WILL feel a greater sense of aliveness. Yes, it starts with the physical, but quite soon after you will realise that you feel calmer, more in control, more harmonious in your thoughts and feelings, and you might even find yourself singing for no apparent reason (I kid you not!). This is simply a knock-on effect from the joy and equilibrium that your body is starting to experience through being fed the foods that suit it best. Again, simple... but *profound*.

If you eat at least half of your diet raw for a week (and make sure the cooked foods are "healthy" – e.g. not fried, roasted or microwaved and as pure as you can get them), then by the end of the first week you will undoubtedly feel the difference physically, emotionally and mentally, and you may well have lost a couple of pounds, or more.

Once you have had your first experience of life on raw, you won't need me or anyone else to explain why it's so easy to get excited and passionate about it! The results simply speak for themselves and you'll know how it feels first-hand; then it's up to you to decide exactly what you want to do with that. This book will show you how.

★ BONUS GOODIES

Download "50 Great Reasons to Go Raw" and "Go Raw For a Day!" at **www.RawFoodBonuses.com**.

Still want more?

Here's a list of the benefits I have experienced and others have shared with me:

- **Feeling good** in your own skin.
- **Feeling lighter** in body, mind and soul.
- **Feeling more connected** to yourself and the world around you.
- **Feeling more purposeful**, clear and divinely guided.
- **Gaining two hours** in your day – or more.
- **Having more love and patience** with others, especially the children!
- **Knowing and really "getting"** that there is a deep wisdom and power in raw, natural plant foods.
- Feeling as if you have **tapped into something magical**.
- Feeling as if you can now **discover and pursue your life purpose**.
- Feeling as if **life is worth living again**.
- **Not minding what others say** because it feels so right.
- Being **committed to your own truth**.
- **Knowing there is wonder and joy** in being "different".
- **Developing an intoxicating fascination** and love of your journey and the energy and power unfolding inside you.
- Trusting that your instincts, if you listen to them, will direct you to **the perfect body and weight for YOU**.
- **Having the faith and self-respect**/self-love to follow your own path, no matter what your friends, family, partner or colleagues say or do.
- **Falling in love with the new life** that is unfolding before you.
- **Feeling excited by the colourful, brave new world** of raw and living foods.

- **Having hope for great health, happiness** and financial security, feeling that anything and everything is possible.
- **Simply loving being alive, clean and connected!**

Sounds quite attractive really, doesn't it?

Well, these are all yours for the taking. And it all starts with your plate.

So now it's time to talk food.

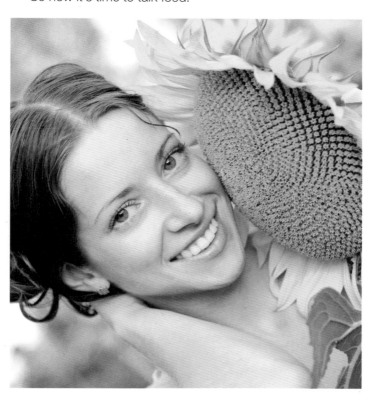

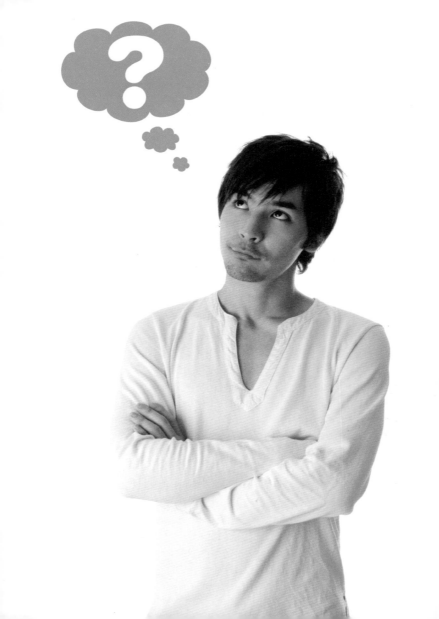

chapter 3
All or nothing?

There's another urban myth about raw food that definitely needs putting straight, and that's that to get the benefits of raw food you need to eat exclusively all raw food or as near to it as possible. Not true. It really doesn't have to be all or nothing.

The fact is, as soon as you start bringing more raw food into your diet (which will likely be displacing some of the cooked food as it does so), you likely will start feeling a difference very quickly.

You're more likely to notice a difference quickly if you are:

- ✪ Aged under 40
- ✪ In "good health"
- ✪ Allowing the less good foods and drinks to fall away
- ✪ Eating according to your appetite (i.e. not overeating)
- ✪ Keeping the raw foods you do eat pure and high water content – mostly fruit and veg

Having said this, these are only guidelines and are not to be taken as definitive as there are many factors that come into play. I have known some people who I would have thought would feel the difference quickly not to, and vice-versa. A lot of it comes down to how clean the overall diet is as well as the raw food component increasing.

For my own part, I was 20 years old when I first dabbled with raw foods. At that point, as I read my first ever raw food book, when I thought about how much raw food I normally ate, I realised it was a rather unimpressive 10% or less – i.e. one piece of fruit per day, if that! I had no clue how I would ever get up to 50% raw, let alone 100% raw (and did I even want to eat all raw? I had no clue, I was just beginning).

However, I found that by bringing raw foods in simply and deliciously – the way I am soon to share with you – I noticed the difference VERY quickly, shockingly so.

Yes, I had youth on my side. However, of those 20 years I had spent 17 of them eating pretty much nothing but junk food. It was not uncommon for me to eat

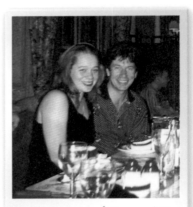

Karen with her father aged 18

chips (fries) twice a day during my late teens when I relied on school canteen food and throwing frozen chips into the deep fat fryer at home. And these would always be accompanied by burgers, sausages or something else meaty. And we mustn't forget the white bread and butter. I really do shudder at the thought of that now, but it tasted good at the time!

Little did I know that a few short years later I would not only find the taste and smell of those things repulsive, but that I would be feeling the way I did when I was a child – energetic, happy and free in my own skin, really and truly ALIVE, literally like I had been reborn – and those feelings came very early on for me in my raw food experiments, despite my junk-food fuelled past.

So, I cannot predict how fast things will change for you, but what I can tell you is this:

- ✪ The more fresh raw food you eat, the better you will look and feel.
- ✪ This is not a race, so always take it at a pace that feels good to you.
- ✪ Clean up the cooked food part of your diet so it doesn't take the shine off the raw.
- ✪ With the raw foods, put your focus on the fresh fruits and veggies – the other foods are great too, but because the fruits and veggies are high water content, they will not only rejuvenate you, but they'll help detoxify you faster too.
- ✪ You'll feel a difference just by increasing the amount of raw food you eat, but to really get a feel for it, you want to tip the balance so that half or more of your diet is raw.

One final note before we address the issue of 100% raw, and this point I cannot stress enough: every step of this journey should feel exciting and fascinating to you. Don't fall into the trap of having this be "another diet" or a "should"... that is not what this is about at all.

Eating raw and living foods is a lifestyle choice, literally a choice between life and… Well, once you start eating more raw, you'll know what it's a choice between.

100% RAW
There's been a lot of talk in raw food circles about the pros and cons of going "all raw" as it's called, over the years.

When I first got into raw food, you could count the number of 100%'ers on one or two hands, so rare were these "god-like" people!

As my own raw food journey progressed and I started meeting other raw foodies, I realised that most people, including myself, were really very happy around the three-quarters mark, which in real terms equates to having a raw breakfast and main meal with the second main meal half-raw and half-cooked, roughly speaking. This is honestly so easy anyone can do it. (I'll be showing you how in Chapter 12).

At 75%–80% raw, which works for most people's lives and preferences, it really is entirely possible to look and feel great (by this point, just a few months in, I had lost about 20 lbs and felt like a brand new Karen). However, what tends to happen is that the better you feel, the more you want to explore how much better it can get! So I set about spending increasing periods of time eating exclusively raw food, and here's what I found...

The energy was AMAZING!

It's at this point that I felt the most profound shifts of all, as if something very powerful was going on that was beyond my total comprehension; that changes were happening on multiple levels in ways that I couldn't fully understand. In fact, some days I felt what can only be described as super-human, as if I could be, do or have anything, and that anything was possible.

Discovering this place and level of aliveness was a huge turning point in my life. Experiencing this first-hand, in my own body, showed me that there are many magical things in life that we can tap into if we do the right things and experiment outside the box.

In some raw food books you will come across stories that will blow your mind – I'm not going to do that just yet as we are just getting started (you can meet some real people with great stories to share later in this book), but take it from me, as fabulous as eating 50% or 75% raw is, when you find a way of eating all-raw that feels really good to you for extended periods of time, you will truly get the meaning of "raw power".

And while this may sound amazing (it is), it's not for everyone. In my work as a raw food coach and teacher working and speaking with literally thousands of raw food enthusiasts, I have found that most people actually do not want to feel that amazing.

It sounds ridiculous I know, but with that level of aliveness and energy comes a new set of challenges, specifically "now what do I do with all this energy?" It is that question and all that goes with that that roughly 75% of my coaching revolves around – quite simply, people are just not used to feeling and looking that good!

So for most people I recommend that you up the amount of raw food at a pace that suits you and then you can acclimatise gradually to the increase in energy – unless you feel ready to really go for it…

That being said, right now we are still at the very beginning. You may be thinking that if that's the downside, then "sign me up!". I truly believe that every man, woman and child walking the earth should have the opportunity to at least try this energy on for size and see where it takes them, because my experience is that it's places most of us never dreamed possible.

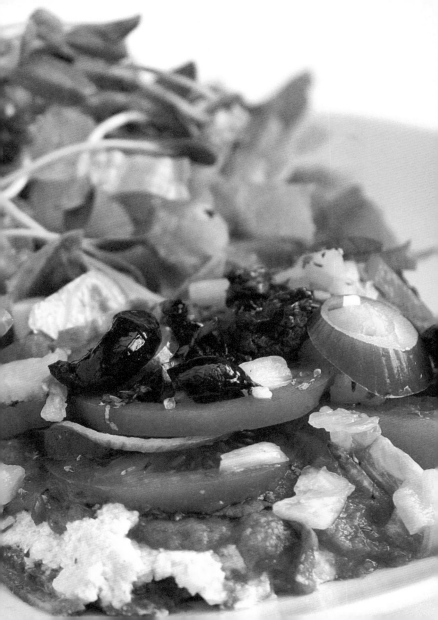

chapter 4
"So what do you eat?"

Possibly THE most commonly asked question of all to any raw foodie is "So what on earth do you eat?"

Some think it's a diet of carrots and apples (and a stick of celery on a "treat" day).

Some think it's all about sushi (and while sushi is raw, most 100% raw foodies are vegetarian or vegan).

Some think it's about eating living creatures (*live* food!) with a few lettuce leaves and a tomato thrown in.

But most people honestly do not have the first clue.

Not surprising, really. I don't know about you, but I certainly wasn't taught about raw food at home or in school. (Home economics as far as I recall was about learning how to make "real lemonade" using fresh lemons and tablespoons of sugar, and how to bake pizza and cookies.)

It really is no wonder that the western world has given birth to generations of wheat and sugar addicts.

So way back when in 1993 I didn't know either. But I was determined to find out and to enjoy the process along the way, and within a few short weeks I was moving and shaking!

Little did I know it then, but my early experiments would later form the foundation of the process that I teach all newbies today.

And that's what I'm about to share with you…

THE RAW INGREDIENTS

There are literally thousands of different raw foods you can enjoy in the world today.

Some come in the form of the staples we have talked about – the "humble" fruits and veggies of which there are hundreds of varieties. Others come in the lesser known food groups such as sprouted foods, sea vegetables and the pretty one in the pack – edible flowers.

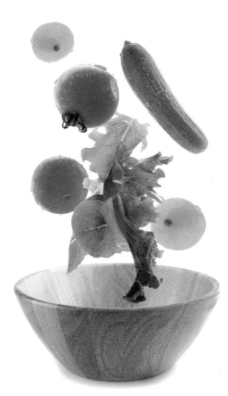

Here follows a complete list of raw food "food groups" – I think you'll be surprised:

- Fresh fruits (apples, pears, pineapple etc.)
- Vegetables (carrots, turnips, sweet potatoes etc.)
- Salad vegetables (tomatoes, bell peppers, cucumbers etc.)
- Leafy green vegetables (kale, watercress, chard etc.)
- Herbs (basil, mint, parsley etc.)
- Wild greens (dandelion, nettle, purslane etc.)
- Nuts (almonds, pine nuts, macadamia nuts etc.)
- Dried fruits (prunes, raisins, sultanas etc.)
- Sprouted beans, pulses and legumes (aduki, mung, lentil etc.)
- Sprouted grains (wheat, rye, barley etc.)
- Seeds (pumpkin, sesame, sunflower etc.)
- Sprouted seeds (quinoa, buckwheat, chia etc.)
- Indoor greens (wheatgrass, sunflower greens, pea shoots etc.)
- Sprouted vegetable seeds (broccoli, mustard, cress etc.)
- Edible flowers (wild rose petals, honeysuckle, lavender blossoms etc.)
- Mushrooms (oyster, portobello, reishi etc.)
- Sea vegetables (dulse, wakame, kelp etc.)
- Algaes (chlorella, spirulina, Klamath lake blue-green algae etc.)
- Oils (olive oil, sesame oil, hemp oil etc.)
- Stimulants (onion, garlic, cayenne pepper etc.)
- Spices (turmeric, cumin, nutmeg etc.)
- Flavourings and sweeteners (cacao, honey, mesquite meal etc.)
- Superfoods (aloe vera, bee pollen, maca etc.)
- Pre-packaged/prepared raw foods (nut butters, seed butters, flax crackers etc.)

As you can see, diversity abounds.

And when you add the different processing methods into the equation, namely...

- Juicing
- Blending
- Milling
- Food processing/homogenising
- Freezing
- Dehydrating
- Marinating
- Fermenting

...it might be easier to begin to get a grasp on the fact that raw food can literally span the entire spectrum of food options – everything from the simplest freshest salad or smoothie, all the way through to a raw gourmet dinner of raw lasagne or pizza or tacos – and more!

21ST CENTURY RAW

When I got into raw food in 1993, there were next to no raw food books in bookstores, next to no recipes in the UK public domain and more recent raw food creations such as raw chocolate bars, potted ice-cream and packets of crackers were still a twinkle in their future creator's eye.

And yet, with all the apparent lack that raw fooding in the early 1990's brought, I honestly had never felt more abundant.

I was gaining in health, energy, happiness, vitality, passion and just about everything that we adults really want. I really did think I had discovered the most amazing life secret (and still do in many respects).

On the flip-side of this new wave of raw food treats,

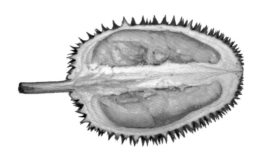

The durian fruit a.k.a. "The King of Fruits".

superfoods and gizmos that we have been blessed with has come something of a double-edged sword – *the raw food recipe book!*

Now, you may not yet have come across one of these, in which case I've caught you just in time! If you have, then what I'm about to say will hopefully bring some peace to your troubled soul.

The truth is raw food recipes books are great – they inspire, make you drool, show what's possible and introduce you to raw ingredients and possibilities that you may never have even considered before.

All good so far.

The downside is that many of these recipe books, in spite of their gifts, also bring overwhelm, confusion and the message that to eat raw food you need to be a world-class chef with the equipment, time, team and budget to match.

Not so.

While yes, having some exceptional and fancy raw food recipes in your repertoire is a wonderful thing and brings diversity, interest and fun to a raw diet, it is totally erroneous to believe that that's what "a raw food diet" is about.

No-one has the time to live like that!

In fact, I don't think I know *anyone* who is overjoyed at the thought of having to buy twenty different ingredients for one recipe and to start prepping a meal four days in advance!

Relieved, then, am I, that when I got into raw food, I had to figure this stuff out for myself.

Without recipe books to inspire or confuse (or scare) and NO previous cooking experience, let alone raw food experience, I simply employed good old fashioned common-sense, experimentation, a sense of play and taste-testing. Before long I had a way of eating raw that not only was quick, easy and delicious, but enabled me to look and feel like that raw food superhero – without even trying.

Furthermore, these results were enjoyed simply off the back of a cheap juicer, blender and hand blender, all costing under £80 (approx. $130 US) and working with extremely limited kitchen space.

Bottom line: If I can do it, anyone can!

Ready to learn the simple secrets to going raw that works?

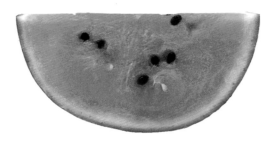

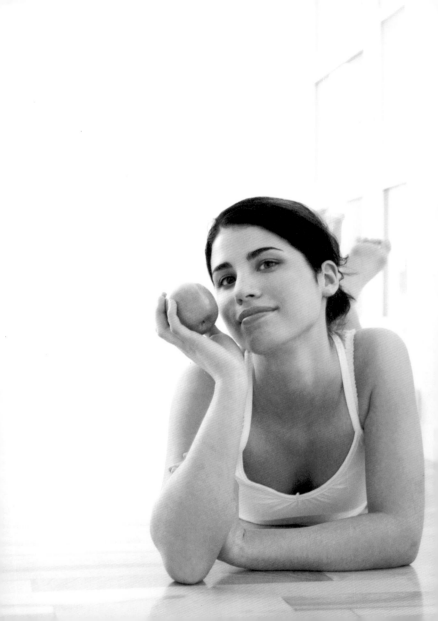

chapter 5
Making the change

Going raw or "more raw" is easy when you know how, and I'm about to show you how.

First of all, it helps to have an idea in mind of how much raw you want to aim for in a typical day. Don't make a big thing about this; keep that all-important sense of play. Tomorrow is another day. It took me FIVE years to be able to stay on 100% raw food for more than a few weeks, so trust me, you have plenty of time to pfaff and fiddle and play with what I'm about to teach you.

On that note, I want and need to mention briefly that in recent years I have noticed a trend where people try and rush the process. While I completely understand why, I also have been around long enough to witness multiple "falling off of wagons", which newbies can take very badly.

My thoughts? *Don't go there!*

While it is not my place to tell you what or what not to do within your own food journey, what I can tell you is that statistically it is only about 1% (or less) of newbies who go raw overnight and stay there without blips – and rather interestingly this 1% are usually very focused, sometimes because of serious illness, or intellectually-driven men! (Generally speaking a woman's journey around food is incredibly different to a guy's. While men tend to find it easier to follow instructions and just get on with it, women tend to have a raft of emotions and stories around food that can take a while to shake. Fret not if this is you; you can find resources and tools to help you via my web site).

So, on the whole my general mantra around transitioning to more raw is "slow and steady wins the race". Unless your life literally depends on it, then I encourage you to use the early days to feel your way through what I'm about to share with you with awareness and lots of positive self-talk and patience, adding to your knowledge and know-how as and when you feel ready. You have the rest of your life to hone your expertise and refine your choices; the honeymoon phase is to be enjoyed and savoured.

With all that said, it *IS* your journey and you will set the pace. What follows now is the easiest, most doable way to bring in more raw food (and drinks) possible. This is how I did it, and I know you will appreciate and value its simplicity as much as I did and continue to, to this very day.

THE EASIEST WAY TO GO RAW

Step 1: Breakfast

Whether you buy into the philosophy that breakfast is the most important meal of the day or not, as far as food choices are concerned, what you eat first in your day will absolutely set the tone for what follows during the rest of the day.

For example, have you ever observed that when you have toast or cereal for breakfast (both wheat-based) that you will tend towards sandwiches for lunch and pasta for your evening meal? (More wheat.) It's not a coincidence.

So, when it comes to going raw, I recommend that you start your day with a totally raw breakfast or as close to it as you can get.

Raw breakfast ideas to get you started:

- Fresh fruit (as much as you want of one type or a combination of fruits as desired)
- Fresh fruit smoothie
- Fruit juice
- Green juice
- Vegetable juice
- Green smoothie
- Almond milk (or other nut milk)
- Banana milk
- Sesame milk (or other seed milk)
- Raw muesli with nut milk
- Dried fruit compote with almond milk
- Fresh fruit salad with or without nut/seed milk

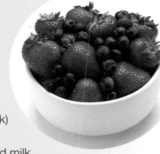

As you can see, your choices are many and varied, and all of these basic recipes, available via **www.TheRawFoodCoach. com**, can be very easily adapted to suit your appetite and palate.

Useful info

According to the ancient Indian philosophy of Ayurveda, the body is in cleansing mode between the hours of 4am and 12 noon. In lay terms this means your body is detoxifying during this eight-hour period and so, to gain maximum benefit from this time, the lighter and purer you can keep your breakfast, the more you will benefit. For those who are looking to lose weight, one of the most powerful things you can do in this regard is to eat or drink only fresh fruits, greens or veggies; anything else will slow the process down and in some cases halt it.

Quantities are not limited. I encourage you and invite you to let your appetite dictate your needs (this is your body's way of speaking to you!). As long as you let your appetite dictate what and when you eat, you will have revelation after revelation about the true desires of your own body and how to reveal your "true" body – your most radiant figure and overall appearance – which may, if you're like most of the population, be hidden underneath layers of superfluous eating.

Bottom line: Breakfast is super-easy and delicious and you can eat this way whether you are at work, home or travelling on the road.

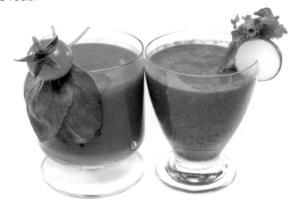

Step 2: Lunch

If you are aiming for 50% raw, then after breakfast it's pretty straightforward: you just make sure that at least half of your plate or glass is made up of raw ingredients. If you're aiming for 75% raw, then you make it three-quarters. No weighing and measuring necessary, just do this by eye.

The easiest way to do this by far (and it's exactly the same for your evening meal) is to make sure that half (or whatever your % is) of your plate comprises of fruit, salad or raw veggies.

This way you get the high-water content foods, which help digest the cooked foods, with their all-important enzymes, and you have the choice of which cooked foods to eat.

When it comes to those cooked foods, as always, I recommend that for maximum benefit and results you go for the clean and "healthy" cooked foods that won't take away too much from the benefits you're gaining from the raw part.

Examples of "healthier" cooked foods that can complement your raw foods:

- Whole-wheat pasta (brown) or other wheat-free pasta alternatives
- Wholegrain rice (brown)
- Organic wholemeal bread, tortillas and rolls (with minimal added ingredients)
- Rye bread or pumpernickel
- Sprouted wheat bread (if you can find a raw brand, so much the better)
- Steamed, boiled or baked yams/sweet potatoes/squash
- Steamed, boiled or baked vegetables of any kind
- Boiled organic potatoes
- Baked organic potatoes with skins
- Minimally processed veggie burgers, sausages etc. (must be free from hydrogenated oils)
- Organic vegetarian cheese, preferably raw (unpasteurised)
- Dairy-free yoghurts or "live" yoghurts without sugar
- Steamed/boiled buckwheat/bulgur wheat/millet/couscous
- Free-range eggs
- Hummous
- Soup
- Stir-fry

chapter 5 Making the change

50%–75% raw lunch ideas to get you started:

- Salad of choice with wholemeal pitta bread
- Salad sandwiches
- Hummous and salad on wholegrain bread of choice
- Baked potato with avocado or raw-slaw filling
- Baked potato with filling of choice and large salad
- Hummous and crudités
- Soup and salad
- Rice salad
- Pasta salad
- Couscous salad
- Cheese salad
- Boiled potatoes coated with olive oil, crushed garlic and fresh basil chopped into a fresh green salad

Again, this is far from rocket science! Even if you work from your desk or car, it is super-easy to pack a lunchbox with everything you need inside of it and enjoy a delicious, healthy and really satisfying lunch.

Useful info

Most people eat lunch because the clock deems it's time. Wherever possible try to resist this habit. Some days you may find that you're hungry at noon; other days you may find you can go as late as 2pm or 3pm. This is normal! Some days we move more than others, thus our calorific needs are higher. The more you relax into eating when your body asks for food, the better you will feel, AND the stubborn weight that was quite possibly being held in place because of eating when NOT hungry is much more likely to disappear!

If your work is office based, consider creating a stash of

raw food goodies and extras in one of your desk drawers. This might include sweet treats like raw snack bars or chocolate bars or trail mix, or it might be the more savoury items for adding to your lunchbox or afternoon nibbles (e.g. nuts, seeds, olives, kale chips etc.).

Bottom line: Lunch has the potential to not just be super-healthy and delicious but actually be MORE enjoyable and varied than what you might be used to. Who knew?

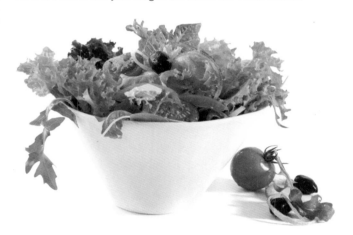

Step 3: Evening Meal

For most people the evening meal is usually eaten at home. If this isn't you, then simply switch my suggestions here with those I gave for lunch. This can still be easy.

Working on the premise that you are preparing and eating at home in the evening, as for lunch, you still want to work to the general % rules to reach your targets, but you probably have a lot more flexibility with your choices. As such you can either have a more elaborate cooked or raw component to your meal because you have the equipment you need right there, but this doesn't have to be the case; it just broadens your options.

50%–75% raw evening meal ideas to get you started:

- Any of the lunch options
- Stir-fry with raw veggies added very last minute
- Veggie burger/sausages with large fresh salad
- Kale salad with chopped potato salad
- Pizza with raw toppings
- Steamed veggies with raw curry sauce
- Roasted veggies with green salad and hummous
- Vine wraps with green salad and hummous
- Cooked beans with chopped fresh salad

Useful info

It is always helpful to eat your evening meal before the sun goes down. This is because our digestive system tends to shut down around the same time meaning that food can hang around longer. This can lead to gas, bloating, heavy stomach or heartburn, not to mention an imperfect sleep and sluggishness on waking.

If it works for you, aim to have lunch be your biggest meal of the day so you can make your evening more enjoyable and expansive. The digestion of food can use up a LOT of energy; far better to use your evenings for creative, leisure, fitness or personal projects than to only be fit for slumping in front of the TV or being ready for bed at 9pm! You WILL have more energy so you better have plans for how to use it!

Bottom line: Just as with lunch, eating high-raw at night is simple, easy and delicious. Just with these simple tweaks that are so easy to implement, you will feel a world of difference. In fact, you won't believe how much and you'll have achieved all this without any feelings of deprivation or sacrifice.

Step 4: Refine & Upgrade Drinks, Snacks & Treats

It's all too easy to think that any eating or drinking outside of the "three square meals" doesn't really count, but of course it does! It all adds up and is very much part of the total picture. Does this mean you have to give up coffee and live on water? Not at all, but it will definitely pay you to keep your mind and taste buds open to other ways of doing this habitual extracurricular consumption.

Focusing on these other choices generally tends to come after a few weeks or months, so is not necessarily something to rush into. I recommend that in the short term you simply

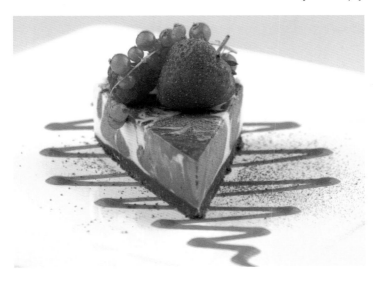

become aware of what you are eating and drinking outside of regular meal times and pay attention to what is driving that choice.

For example, are you drinking coffee because you lack energy? (Raw food can and will take care of this, but caffeine is a drug so you'll need to approach it as such.)

Are you reaching for the chocolate bar because you think you deserve a treat? (I'm sure you do, but what may be a treat for your taste buds may not be such a great treat for your cells! Why not go for the win-win? It's yours for the taking.)

Are you eating dessert every night after your main meal because you think that constitutes "a proper meal"? (Your body loves it when you keep things simple, so desserts don't need to be off the menu, but they do ideally need to have a slot of their own.)

As you gain awareness around these habits and behaviours, you will for sure learn a lot about yourself.

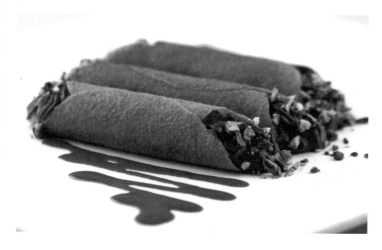

At all times have compassion, patience and know that when you are ready to upgrade, there is a world of healthy and delicious alternatives waiting for you. Some of these we have discussed already; many can be found in your local health food shop or raw food online store or at your nearest raw food café or restaurant. (Both of the delicious desserts featured in this chapter are 100% raw – what *could* you be missing out on?!)

Raspberry Passion Pudding with a slice of Raw Chocolate Torte anyone?

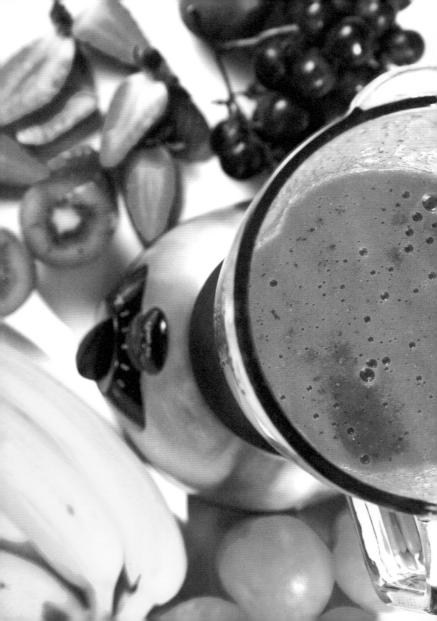

chapter 6
Equipping your kitchen

As mentioned previously, I got started with the most basic and cheapest pieces of kitchen equipment, namely:

- ✪ A centrifugal juicer (one with a spinning/grating disc)
- ✪ A hand-held blender
- ✪ A tabletop blender

All of these stood me in great stead for a number of years, so please don't fall into the all too common trap of thinking that you need to spend hundreds or thousands of pounds or dollars on top-of-the-range kitchen equipment.

Sure, you do get what you pay for and today I wouldn't be without my Champion juicer, Vitamix blender, Excalibur dehydrator and Cuisinart food processor as they are more powerful and durable than cheaper models *BUT* I thrived on my raw diet at the start just as well as I do today – simple almost always is better.

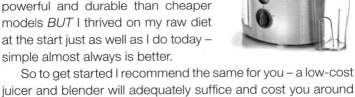

So to get started I recommend the same for you – a low-cost juicer and blender will adequately suffice and cost you around £50 (approx. $75 US) for both. In fact you might even find them for a complete steal via a local second-hand outlet or eBay. The hand blender is not necessary; I just bought one of those because it was super-cheap and I'd read about it in a book! It does, however, serve as a great in-between gadget if you don't have a food processor and is very handy for travelling, especially if you find a battery-operated model.

If you *do* have cash to invest, then a food processor would be my next recommendation with the dehydrator (an oven-like piece of equipment that dries but doesn't bake) the last on the list, because as handy as it is, it does tend to complicate things and can definitely contribute towards that sense that raw food is difficult or time-consuming, neither of which, as we have discussed extensively, need to be true.

In Chapter 14 I'm sharing with you 15 of my own personal favourite raw food recipes. All of these are quick, easy and delicious and the only electrical item you need is a blender. Literally 5–10 minutes and you'll be done. Cooking by comparison seems like a big waste of time to me now, honestly.

If you're a busy person (and who *isn't* these days?), then you will love how much time you save in the kitchen and how much time you gain in energy. The two gains combined easily equate to an extra 2½ hours per day.

When it comes to purchasing your kitchen equipment, for the cheaper items your local electrical store or even supermarket can suffice. See **www.TheRawFoodDirectory.com** for the more expensive items you'll likely need to order online.

SETTING YOURSELF UP FOR SUCCESS

I truly believe that when you start putting healthier and cleaner foods into your body, you soon start wanting your *kitchen* to reflect your new-found sparkle! For this reason I recommend that you take half a day or more to detox your kitchen and keep in it only the foods that you are happy to put in your body.

If you are sharing your kitchen with someone who has different ideas, no worries, just let them know that you're spring cleaning and suggest that you have your own separate "zones" where you can do your thing and they can do theirs. It's highly unlikely that they will object – everyone loves having their own territory.

On a practical level, it definitely pays to give your fridge, freezer and cupboards a good scrub and clean. This is as much symbolic as it is hygienic. When you are done, you will literally feel the difference inside and out, and your commitment to yourself will be palpable.

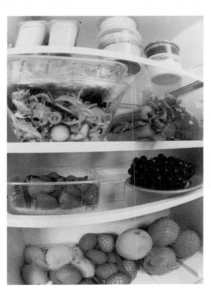

When it comes to experiencing a raw high, I have learned time and again that the days I feel the most amazing and alive are those when I couple eating super-clean and light (all raw) with radically cleaning and sorting my home. I love it!

I encourage you to try this for yourself... you really will feel like a new person and you'll feel a sense of order, peace and possibility that you may not have felt for a very long time.

It's Time to Get Rawganized!

Bear in mind that in this book we are simply getting you started, so I'm not about to go into a whole kitchen transformation teach-in with you (if you're ready for that then my "Let's Get Rawganized!" program is the most comprehensive system for setting yourself up for raw success imaginable), but chances are that if you've got this far or have already started dabbling with raw food, then you will be ready for more. In which case, aside from the equipment purchasing and kitchen detoxing, I encourage you to start creating your "Rawganized Kitchen Binder" right away.

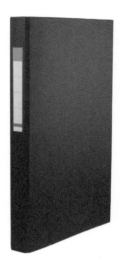

Creating your binder is super-easy and you'll adore it, I promise. To get yours going, simply find yourself a robust metal-ring binder (preferably one that you find beautiful), some divider tabs (a 10-part set is perfect) and some clear hole-punched plastic sleeves (20+ is great) to file in your binder. These form the basis of your binder.

Next, print out the free bonuses that come to you with this book (download yours online at **www.RawFoodBonuses.com**), hole punch them and add them to your binder. I recommend that you slip the recipe pages into the clear plastic sleeves, as this will protect them from damage and spills.

Already you have the start of a fabulous Rawganized Binder!

Next step, go to **www.TheRawFoodCoach.com** and print off any other raw information sheets and recipes that you can lay your hands on – you'll find these under FREE STUFF and also dotted around the site in different places. Add these to your binder.

Finally, as you progress in your raw food journey, get together any other raw food recipes, magazine cuttings, mail order catalogues and so forth and hole-punch or plastic-sleeve those too. In no time at all you'll have a resource that will prove invaluable to you from this moment forward – something I wish I had had way back when I got started. (If you want a Rawganized binder that's packed with information from the start, "Let's Get Rawganized!" will be a godsend. Full details at **www.LetsGetRawganized.com**.)

Now You're Rawganized!

The right equipment, a clean and detoxed kitchen and a Rawganized Binder really are the three most important things you can take care of as you start your journey into raw food. Very soon you'll realise that as your inner and outer environments transform and upgrade, you'll have the clarity, energy and vitality to start making other life changes come true also...

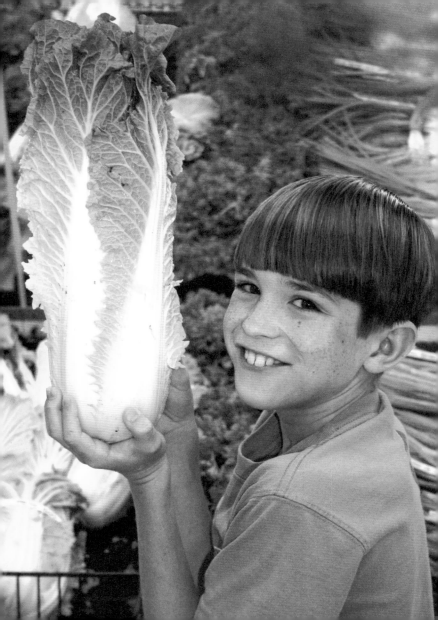

chapter 7
Raw shopping

Wherever you live in the world, chances are that you will have far greater access to quality raw foods than you currently know.

Most of us have become very reliant on supermarkets for both variety and convenience, and you will find that they may still cater pretty well for a radiant raw diet, but there's also a good chance that you will need to cast your net a little wider in order to get the best produce and the sweetest treats.

On the following pages you'll find a brief overview of the various different shopping options available to you. Some will be obvious; others may be new to you. Either way, I invite you to pick at least one of those that you haven't ventured inside before and check it out. A whole new world of food and experience literally could be opened right up to you.

Here's what we're going to be looking at:

- Supermarkets
- Health food shops
- Wholefood warehouses
- Specialist food shops, including Asian and Oriental
- Farmers markets
- Local markets
- Local greengrocers

- Organic box deliveries
- Pick-your-own
- Farm shops
- Roadside stalls
- Mail order companies

SUPERMARKETS

There's no doubt about it that for most people, supermarkets are the most convenient place to shop.

Everything all in one place – just park, shop and go. Internet shopping and home delivery also has its obvious benefits, such as not needing to queue or physically do the shop yourself, and being able to have what you want more often than not, rather than finding empty selves. However, although convenient, there are ethical concerns to bear in mind, with the bulk-buying ability of supermarkets and low wages often making vast sums of money for the privileged few, all the while treating food as a commodity, rather than something which feeds the body and soul of the local population. That said, as supermarkets continue to compete against each other, the quality and diversity of foods continues to improve, and prices can be competitive also.

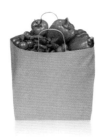
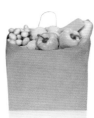
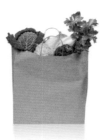

HEALTH FOOD SHOPS

Health food shops vary enormously. If you can find a good one, which believes that good health comes from good food rather than aisles of supplements and packets, so much 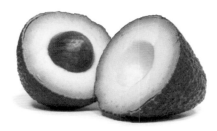 the better. There are now even chains of health food shops like this, such as *Whole Foods Market*. True health food stores often have a wonderful atmosphere and the vitality of the produce on display is positively magnetic! The downside of these stores is often the price tag unfortunately. They don't yet have the bulk buying ability of the conventional supermarkets, or if they do, then it's simply about buying better quality produce or paying the farmers more money – a good thing, so as with most pricier things in life, you often get the quality that you pay for.

WHOLEFOOD WAREHOUSES

These are more often suppliers of dried and bottled foods, such as wholegrains, nuts, beans, seeds, tahini and the like. If you use a lot of these foods (and ideally you should to complement the fresh fruit and vegetables), then this could prove to be a very cost efficient way of buying, especially if you can buy in bulk with a friend or group and split the costs. Often these types of outlets have strong ethics and are run as a co-operative, so prices and values are often excellent, making for a happier, more satisfying shopping experience all round.

SPECIALIST FOOD SHOPS, INCLUDING ASIAN AND ORIENTAL

As you begin to explore the wide range of raw foods available to you, you may very well find yourself drawn to different types of shops. Asian shops often house a wonderful treasure trove of dried herbs, spices, nuts and seeds, and import the most wonderful Pakistani mangoes in the summer. while oriental shops are well known for exotic fruits, such as the durian, jackfruit, young coconuts (pictured) and large papaya, amongst many other hard to find delicacies.

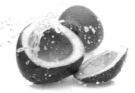

FARMERS MARKETS

In the UK and across America, farmers markets are springing up with more and more regularity, providing an ever-changing vista of the freshest produce available, second only to growing your own.

Farmers from the local region, or in some cases, from all over the country, bring their produce to market on a set day of the week or month, and sell at remarkably low prices to the health conscious, who know that fresh is best. Often these are organic farmers, who truly love their work and talking about the fruits of their labours – you often come away with as much fascinating information as you do produce, making the experience a truly nourishing one.

LOCAL MARKETS

Traditional markets tend to sell non-organic fresh fruit and vegetables, but at very cheap prices. This is fine if you are experimenting, or if money is very tight, but long term is not the best option, as the produce is often past its best, or about to be, and has not been farmed or distributed with a great deal of TLC. Now and again you may find a genuine bargain, with produce riper and more succulent than your local supermarket, so don't rule out the possibility altogether, but bear in mind that this tends to be the exception rather than the rule – it really depends where you are in the world. Occasionally you will find a market seller who operates in the same way as a local greengrocer (see below), which is a real coup!

LOCAL GREENGROCERS

Greengrocers also vary, depending on the standards of the owner. Some greengrocers may obtain produce from the same outlets as the market sellers, while others may make regular trips to a major city to pick up the freshly imported produce. It's worth visiting a few in your area to get a feel for the staff and the quality of produce, as all greengrocers are not equal. If you find a good one, stick with them, give them your support, and even make suggestions if it seems appropriate. These kinds of establishments thrive on the one-to-one contact with their customers, and realise that what you want is likely what others also want. If you find yourself buying a large amount of produce at a time, why not ask if you can order in bulk for a discount? Chances are they will say yes, and also, you may find that they deliver as well.

ORGANIC BOX DELIVERIES

Box schemes can work in one of two ways – either you receive a standard box containing pre-decided produce depending on what's in season, or you can select your own, paying by weight or unit, again, usually depending on what's in season. There are many different companies to choose from these days, both local and nationwide, so if this is an option which appeals to you and you have a bad experience with one, do not assume that all companies are the same. These companies tend to specialise in local or seasonal produce, so sometimes choice may be limited, but again, do some homework (the internet is usually the best way to find out), and you may find the perfect solution for you.

PICK-YOUR-OWN

Typically non-organic (unfortunately), pick-your-own outlets provide many a fun summer's afternoon, spent amongst the berry bushes. Costs are lower because of the fact you are providing the labour, and also you get to choose exactly the food you do and don't want, which is very gratifying, but of course, at the back of your mind is the question, "How much pesticide has been sprayed on these?"

Aside from this issue, however, is the fact that food doesn't come much fresher than this, and it's wonderful to be out in the open air, selecting your next meal or desserts. Hopefully in the future more and more organic farms will offer this service.

FARM SHOPS

Farm shops are one-step removed from pick-your-own, because the picking has already been done for you, and usually the produce has been picked the same day, or just a few hours before you arrived. Farm shop produce is renowned for being excellent value for money, providing truly delicious fresh and vibrant produce, and more and more organic farms are offering this service now.

ROADSIDE STALLS

In some parts of the country you may find a table of produce outside someone's home, or hidden down an alley, and you may find some excellent bargains along the way. Often grown by the householder, they find they have a surplus and display for passers-by to take advantage of, going on trust that the produce will be paid for as ticketed. As with local greengrocers and box schemes, the quality of the produce is bound to vary from vendor to vendor, but there's no doubt that some bargains can be picked up this way, and of course there's the novelty of surprise! The only drawback is, of course, if you find a food you like, it may not be there again for a while, if ever!

MAIL ORDER COMPANIES

Possibly the best answer to today's fast-paced lifestyle, mail order companies are waiting to take your call often around the clock. Internet-based ones are there displaying their wares 24/7, so you can browse for as long as you wish, change your order as many times as you wish, and pay without queuing.

The other main benefit of this route is that you can print off lists, compare prices between sites, often write messages to the company expressing preferences, questions or suggestions, and the good thing for most people is that goods ordered this way often come within a day or so, direct to the delivery address of your choice. The downsides to this are that the packaging isn't always environmentally friendly, orders can sometimes be picked wrong, and you sometimes don't know 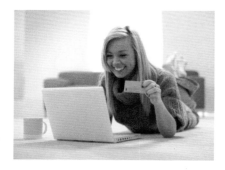 in advance what's out of stock, but for most people the benefits outweigh the drawbacks, and mail order is proving more and more popular.

So these are your options. If you've found more – terrific! Most importantly, whether you are new to raw food or are a longer-term enthusiast, make sure you keep your mind and body open to new foods on a regular basis. Discovering a new food that you love is always a great thing at any stage of your journey.

Why not check out a new option today?

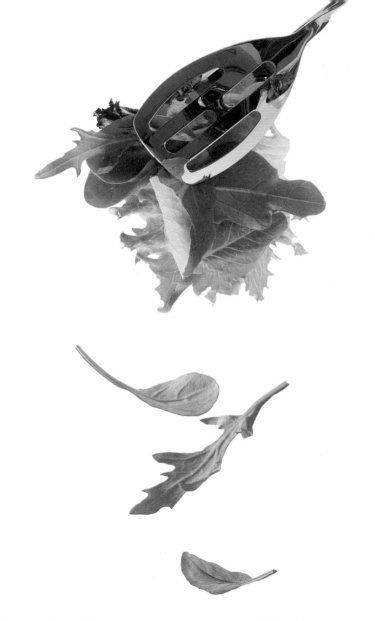

chapter 8
Raw food nutrition

One of the most common questions raised around eating raw is about whether it's nutritionally sound, i.e. "Can you get everything that you need from a raw food diet?"

The answer is yes, you can, if you make a point of eating a well-rounded and diverse, high quality diet, which we'll discuss further in a moment.

There are also some other important factors that need to be taken into account regarding how *your* unique body processes food, ranging from your body type, to your dietary and medical history, your metabolism, your genetics, your current lifestyle and emotional state and much more, and so even though people would absolutely love for it to be the case, there really *isn't* a one-size-fits-all answer.

First of all, know that whatever diet you eat, the amount of nutrition that you gain from your food is *not* specifically about what or how much you eat, but about how well you can *assimilate and absorb* the nutrients you take in. For some people with particularly poor digestive functioning, this can be much less than what they actually put into their body, so if you can't seem to gain weight or thrive no matter what you eat, then it's worth being checked out professionally to see if you have absorption issues or whether it's just a case of needing to modify your diet.

The second important issue as mentioned is to make sure that you eat a wide variety of raw foods and the highest quality possible. This means foods from all the different food groups spread over a week or month, going for organic wherever possible, eating a whole spectrum of different colours of the rainbow and eating seasonally and locally wherever possible. This ensures nutritional diversity as well as simply (but just as importantly) getting more joy and pleasure from your food. And while some people find that they can thrive on a raw vegan diet with no animal products featuring at all, others find they can eat vegan for a while, but for them personally it's not sustainable for the long term. If you are considering going vegan as well as eating more raw, you will have to experiment to see which group you fall into if you don't know already.

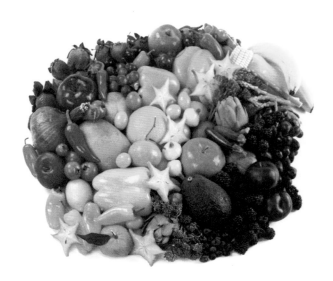

The third critical factor that I really must include is about the importance of mindset. One of the things I have learned over the years from working and speaking with literally thousands of people in this arena is that as much as the very real nuts-and-bolts of nutrition play a huge part in our health and well-being, the way we think and feel about what we are eating also plays an enormous part. Although not tangible or measurable, my observations suggest that absolutely the way that people approach their diet is a *huge* influence on the results they get. For this reason I have always approached any dietary change of my own with enthusiasm, optimism and excitement and yet have retained an open and flexible mind so I can easily and unemotionally tweak or overhaul my diet if and when necessary.

On looking at how others have or haven't thrived when making a diet change I can always see, as I'm sure you can too if you think about it, a direct correlation between how they *feel* about that change and the results they experience. The mind and body are intimately and powerfully inter-connected, and both influence each other phenomenally. For this reason I recommend that you only make changes to your diet that you can genuinely believe in and can get really excited about; otherwise, your mind will be at conflict with your body, which is never fun, no matter how healthfully you may be eating!

Now, before we move on to some raw nutrition facts, there's one final point I need to make, which always makes me smile. One of the ironies about the whole "can raw food give you everything you need?" question is, of course, that when we're busy eating junk food full-time like many of us have such great experience with, rarely do we stop to ask ourselves if we are getting enough nutrition from *that* diet, and yet as soon as we clean up our act and start paying attention to what we eat and eat *superior* foods rather than nutritionally-deficient ones, suddenly we

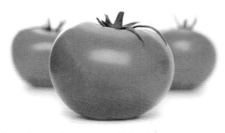

worry that we are going to miss out on something!

Although it *is* ironic, it's still wise to pay attention because wherever we are starting from we have a foundation from which to measure our results. I have seen people literally look ten years younger after a few months on raw food and I have seen some people look like they have aged ten years. The difference between the two is usually the quality and diversity of raw foods they are eating (and if they are eating enough) and also, as discussed, how well they are absorbing what they eat and the way in which they are mentally and emotionally embracing what they are doing.

With this in mind, my advice is simple. Keep your mind and actions positive, stay flexible and open-minded in your approach, and providing you keep checking in with yourself and monitoring what works and what doesn't, you should find it very easy to find the perfect balance for you.

WHY RAW FOOD ROCKS

Imagine taking a humble nut, bean or seed, cooking it and then planting it in the ground and watering it. Will it grow? No, of course not – it's now technically an enzymatically "dead" food and can no longer grow or reproduce itself, but it can still give you some degree of nourishment and become a source of fuel for you.

Imagine now taking a second nut, bean or seed that *hasn't* been cooked and doing exactly the same thing. Will it grow this time? Absolutely – unless it has been damaged in some other way, and not only that, when it does grow, its nutrition will increase by up to several hundred or even thousand per cent in just a few short days!

You see, when you eat sprouted foods such as nuts, beans, seeds and grains, not only does your body receive a massive amount of nutrition from a very small amount of food, but it also receives a whole raft of things that it could not ever receive from its cooked counterpart, including oxygen, phytonutrients, enzymes, a much higher amount of vitamins, minerals and water, plus a whole number of things that modern science is only just starting to name and quantify.

What's important to know here is that, as valuable as it is, nutrition as we know it is a very new science of just a few decades standing. Many argue, myself included, that while we have made huge strides in our scientific understanding of food, there is still a very long way to go.

Never is this more apparent than when studying raw food, as you will experience for yourself, and that's because not only are you dealing with "live" food, but when you start eating more raw foods you become aware very quickly that you are benefiting from way more of something than most scientists are able to measure or give a name to.

The fact is you start to feel better very

quickly in ways both subtle and obvious, and it becomes clear just as quickly that there is far more at play here than simply increased nutrition.

One of my favourite mentors and health educators of all time is the esteemed Dr Brian Clement of the Hippocrates Health Institute in Florida. Dr Clement has been working with clients and seriously ill people from all around the world since the 1970's when he trained with "The Mother of Living Foods", Dr Ann Wigmore. As both a medic and a scientist, Dr Clement has made it part of his life's work to shed light on why raw and living foods are so incredibly powerful and beneficial to the body and he talks extensively about this in his books, but in summary of the brilliance that Dr Clement has to teach, there's one area of his work that I want to share with you to begin to illustrate what we really are tapping into when we "liven up" our diet.

Back in the 1990's Dr Clement decided to work with a cutting-edge scientist to investigate the auric field of various different foods to see exactly how what we eat impacts on us energetically. The fact is, even though we see ourselves as very "real" human beings, as with everything in this universe, including our food, what we truly are is a bundle of energy that appears in a solid form. Dr Clement decided to use Kirlian photography, a special type of photography that captures the energy field around a person or object, to gain deeper insight into the energy fields of different foods and how they affect us when we ingest them. What he discovered was absolutely fascinating.

Dr Clement discovered that natural raw foods such as fresh fruits, vegetables and living foods such as wheatgrass, sunflower greens and sprouted foods, have a beautiful colourful aura around them, indicating vitality and a good, strong, healthy

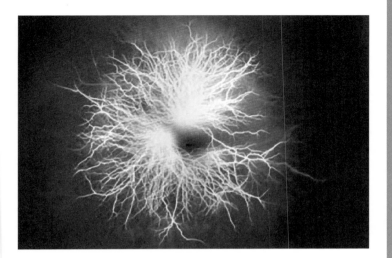

energy. Conversely he saw that junk foods, and in the case he shared with me, a hamburger, had a dark, much smaller energy field around it. Aside from the obvious, which I feel speaks for itself, further investigation showed that when a person went to eat the fast-food, their own auric field would shrink and darken in response to the food that was coming in and would continue to do so once eaten, and conversely when they ate raw and living foods, their aura expanded and got brighter.

For myself, being someone who is sensitive to energy and also intuitive, I truly believe that this type of investigation into food holds as much, if not more, value than the conventional intellectual analysis of food. And although we may still be years away from viewing our food energetically in mainstream science, what's for sure is that we can all start experiencing the benefits and the awareness of this for ourselves first-hand, right here, today.

RAW SCIENCE

While Dr Clement's work is brilliant and fascinating, what about the more mainstream scientific facts about raw food? What's out there, and if it's so compelling, why aren't more people eating more raw?

This is a good question and one I've been asked many times. The fact is there is a lot of science in existence to support eating more raw foods, but sadly it is rarely publicised or supported because there's very few people or organisations that are prepared to fund it.

And while we can't go into a whole lot of detail here in this chapter because of space, I'd like to share with you here details of one particularly thought-provoking study that gives us all some serious food for thought.

The study in question, an extensive one indeed and often referred to as "Pottenger's Cats", was created and led by Dr Francis M. Pottenger between 1932 and 1942, involving 900 cats over four generations. The study, which was effectively to see the difference between feeding a cat a raw diet versus a cooked one, was initiated because Pottenger had witnessed significant differences in the health and behaviour of cats quite by chance when circumstance led him to feed the cats in his laboratory a raw diet rather than the usual cooked one. Without even expecting any differences to occur, he noticed that the improvement in all of the cats being fed raw meat and milk was too marked and fascinating to ignore, and so it was that Dr Pottenger decided to investigate more thoroughly and to perform a controlled experiment to verify these facts scientifically.

Over the decade that the study was carried out, the cats were divided into seven different groups. Two of the groups were fed raw milk and meat in different ratios, one group ate cooked meat and consumed raw milk, and the other four groups were fed raw meat and consumed cooked milk in various different forms to see what difference that would make.

In the groups receiving raw milk and raw meat it was found that they were well-formed cats with good bone structure, a broad dental arch (ensuring healthy teeth formation), their nasal cavities were adequate, they had no evidence of infection or parasites and they behaved in a predictable manner. In reproductive terms they reproduced normally from one generation to the next and were able to nurse successfully.

All of the cats who were part of the five groups featuring cooked meat *or* milk came to demonstrate poor health and poor social/emotional habits very quickly.

In the case of the cats receiving cooked meat, in the first generation roughly one-quarter aborted. In the second generation, about 70% aborted live births. Many cats died in labour having great difficulty with delivery, and the mortality rate of the kittens was high. Mothers could not lactate and the

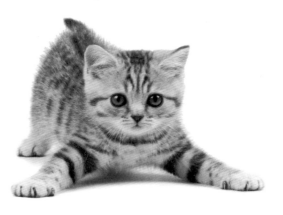

kittens were often too weak to nurse. The skeletal pattern of the kittens was also different to the norm with longer, narrow faces. Also, their teeth did not come through at the regular time and diseases of the gums developed. By the third generation the cats' bones were fine and weak, with small and irregular teeth. The females expressed increased irritability and aggression, while the males became more docile and unaggressive. Interest in sex interest was slack or perverted. Skin lesions, allergies and intestinal parasites became increasingly worse from one generation to another. Pneumonia, diarrhoea, arthritis and many other degenerative conditions seen in humans became apparent.

There was no fourth generation in any of the processed food groups because either the third generation parents were sterile or the fourth generation cats died before birth.

Finally, and rather interestingly, Dr Pottenger discovered that it took *four* generations on raw meat and raw milk to bring the kittens of second-generation degenerating cats back to normal.

Granted, we are not cats, but it is not difficult to see that here in the twenty-first century we are experiencing unprecedented levels of infertility, disease and mental and emotional health issues. In fact Dr Pottenger himself is purported to have said, *"While no attempt will be made to correlate the changes in the animals studied with malformations found in humans, the similarity is so obvious that parallel pictures will suggest themselves."*

THE PROOF OF THE PUDDING...

Whatever we choose to believe about food, science or nutrition, our own first-hand experience is ultimately our greatest litmus test. Studies can be skewed, false assumptions made and results misinterpreted – and that's not even taking into consideration the many variables, constituent parts and possibilities that any experiment comprises.

When it comes to nutrition, your body, your health and ultimately your happiness, I firmly believe that you have to give anything you're trying your best, unbiased shot… and then see for yourself. Your body has no reason to lie, and whatever you learn about yourself in the process of experimentation can only be a gain.

I feel certain that providing you use your common sense, eat a wide variety of raw foods and keep paying attention as you go, you'll start noticing some very real and impressive differences when you increase the amount of raw food in your diet.

In fact, if you're anything like the thousands of people I have communicated with over the past two decades, it could only be a matter of days before you begin to notice that every aspect of yourself is waking up and starting to operate from a very different level of experience and vitality… and each time you return to your old ways you will experience the opposite just as acutely!

What will you choose?

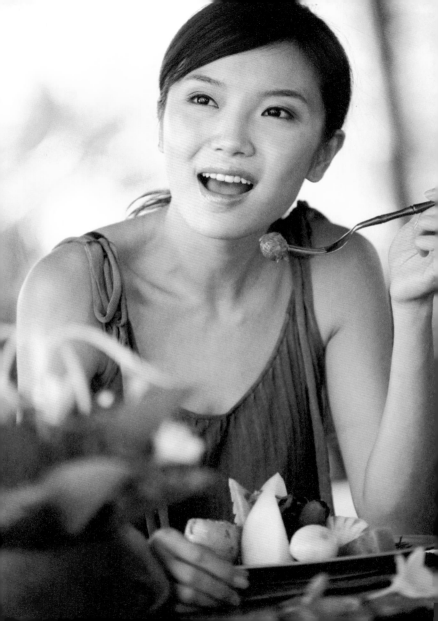

chapter 9
Family & social situations

HOW TO EXPLAIN YOUR FOOD CHOICES TO FRIENDS AND FAMILY

If you decide to eat more raw food, then saying that you are "going raw" or have "gone raw" to your nearest and dearest may be easy or challenging depending on a) what they're used to seeing you eat, and b) what they themselves eat.

For this reason I recommend that in the early days, if you are not sure what a response is likely to be or you suspect it won't be helpful, that you say something like "I'm dabbling with eating more fresh foods" or "I'm on a detox", or something similar that you feel comfortable with that will explain any food choices you make that seem out of character.

The word "raw" generates such different responses from people that, unless you know your friends and family will be supportive of you, it's probably best that you use terms like "fresh", "organic", "whole" or "natural" – all of these are a good fit, but they don't sound as intense as "raw", and the level of interest won't be quite so intense either! You'll be glad you kept it low key, especially when you are still finding your feet.

Also remember that when it comes to food, everyone has an opinion and we all think we're right (or even if we don't, we still tend to defend what we eat, so emotive is this subject). So do what you want to do, make it easy for yourself, especially in the early days and don't push it on anyone. That way they won't push back and you can eat what you want in peace.

Here follow my top tips for navigating those waters otherwise known as explaining your choices to your family for the first time, or even the umpteenth!

1 **Keep it simple.** A long conversation is usually not necessary; this is not world politics and you are not changing gender or adopting a child. You are simply changing the way you are eating, and it doesn't have to affect them at all, after all they are not the one eating it!

2 **Keep calm.** You may be congratulated or challenged. It can go either or both ways. Whichever way it goes, it is up to you to be calm and unfettered by it. Opinions are opinions; they do not have to dictate your life or your own opinions.

3 **Stay focused.** You chose to eat more raw for a reason (or many reasons); remain aware of what those reasons are at all times. The more you have and the more they make sense, the more likely others will understand and admire you.

4 **Keep your opinions to yourself.** In your new incarnation as a raw food fan, you may well find yourself wanting to "spread the word" – rarely a good move. This is often the quickest way to turn what could be a simple and stress-free conversation into a full-scale food debate, or worse! Don't do it.

5 **Only say more if asked.** As per above, the less you say, generally the better. When you do say more, have it be in response to someone's (polite) question. Keep it light and definitely non-confrontational and non-judgemental. Not doing so is the quickest way to make people turn against the concept of raw food, and then, possibly, you!

6 **Impress, wow and seduce.** Whether you are discussing

food, serving it or bringing it along, be sure to present your best and most favourite recipes. This is not the time to say that a simple salad does it for you, even if it's the truth. They won't believe you and they won't want to try it either. Bring on the raw chocolate cake and the strawberry "cheezecake" and it could well be a very different story!

7 **Relax**. There is nothing more off-putting, unattractive and unconvincing than sitting with someone who is uptight and regimental about their food choices. Be cool. If you eat something that's not raw or as healthy as you'd like, just roll with it in whatever way works for you. Laugh. Chat. Be yourself. Let the food fall into the background and be the supporting role in your life, not the main focus, and others will see you rather than your plate.

I hope these tips help as you go forward into your first social interactions, but remember, ultimately it is up to you to know your own circles and what way of handling things is most appropriate. Humour and brevity tend to work well in most situations, especially with families.

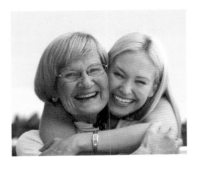

Be prepared to laugh at yourself if necessary. Not everyone will understand your reasoning, and that's okay. There may be many things about them that you don't understand or agree with either, and that's okay too.

Live and let live, and you will find that others will extend you the same courtesy.

EATING RAW IN RESTAURANTS

One of the most common questions I get asked is, "How do you eat raw in a restaurant?" To which I reply, "Very easily, most

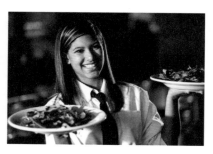

of the time!" and it's true. Eating out does not have to be difficult; you just have to know a few key tricks and put them into practice when you need to, and they will serve you time and again.

What also helps is knowing what you like. I love the classic avocado, tomato and cucumber mix, so if I can get this in generous portions served on a bed of fresh green leaves with some lemon squeezed on top, then generally I am a very happy customer! For this reason you might find it a good idea to draw up a list of your favourite (common) raw foods and create some simple salad combinations from them – six would be great – and have them on hand to use when ordering, or even to give to the waiter so he can pass them to the chef.

Tips for ordering raw food successfully in a restaurant

- ✪ If you're very unfamiliar with a restaurant or simply want to be clued up, check the restaurant's web site or call them in advance for a copy of the menu.
- ✪ If you call them in advance with questions or requests, they are more likely to cater for you because you've given them notice.
- ✪ Scan the entire menu first to get a handle on what ingredients are in the kitchen.

✪ Decide what your ideal meal will be, based on a main dish already on the menu (usually a salad) and with other ingredients added and any that you don't want taken away.

✪ If you keep it as a straight swap (remove cheese, replace with avocado), most restaurants are fine with this because it's simple and easy to manage in every way; it's when you want to add other things and the meal gets out of proportion to the original dish (adding more than you're taking away) that some waiting staff can get confused or feel overwhelmed because they don't know what to do about pricing. This is why I approach this in stages; at the very least we get the straight swap – anything else is a bonus.

Some common and usually easy-to-order raw meals/sides:

✪ Tomato and basil salad
✪ Gazpacho (tomato-based raw soup)
✪ Fruit salad
✪ Melon plate
✪ Crudités and guacamole
✪ Basic salad
✪ Additions of:

Olives
Grated carrot
Grated beetroot
Orange slices
Nuts
Broccoli florets
Cauliflower florets

Cucumber spears
Apple slices
Pineapple chunks
Mango slices
Lemon slices
Fresh herbs
Additional greens
Olive oil & lemon dressing

How to Get What You Want

There are really two vital things to have a handle on when it comes to ordering in a restaurant, and these are:

✪ Attitude
✪ Know-how

Attitude comes first because it really begins and ends with that; it's vital that you enter into any social eating situation with a positive attitude, otherwise, it is going to be uphill all the way, and can lead to a whole catalogue of frustrations and even ruin an occasion. In all my years of eating raw I have found that the best possible attitude to go into a non-raw restaurant situation is a combination of the following:

✪ Light-hearted
✪ Focused but flexible
✪ Humorous
✪ Polite
✪ Grateful
✪ Open
✪ And being mildly cheeky never hurts either!

I've also found through coaching clients and conversations with fellow raw foodies that others who have adopted this or a similar attitude have always been successful at getting a decent raw meal, while others who have been uptight, intense, resentful or overly-serious have not usually fared as well. The first thing to bear in mind here is that you are not just really ordering for yourself. In many regards you are an ambassador for this "new" way of eating called "raw". How you come across in social situations can actually colour not just your own experience but fellow diners and restaurant staff's perception of those who eat raw. Needless to say, if you go into a restaurant situation with a positive attitude, not only do you usually get what you want, but positive associations are made with "raw food people" – we are all helping each other!

So why the importance in attitude? Well, you will be dealing with real human beings here – either the waiter or the chef, possibly both. If you are clear and prepared, then usually the waiter will be able to handle your order just fine, but if you are making it complicated for them to understand, then one of the chefs, or even the head chef, might be called out. With this in mind, really, you don't want to be asking for any of the raw gourmet dishes you may have seen! Yes, everyone around you might be eating fancy, but most restaurants today really can struggle with even a basic salad in my experience (even the ones you would think could handle it), so now is not the time to make things even more difficult for them – or for you, because chances are that's what it will be.

INTRODUCING RAW FOOD TO YOUR PARTNER OR CHILDREN

In the early days I strongly recommend that you keep your focus on your own food journey and experiments. Of course it's tempting to want to involve your family as soon as possible, especially if you are feeling great benefits and want them to experience the same, but experience tells me that it is far better for you to do your own learning and experiments alone at first and then, when you think you've got it nailed and to a point of consistency and balance, you can look to introducing simple recipes and teachings to your children and other family members.

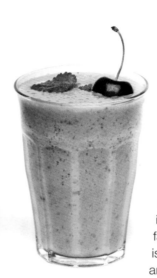

I understand that this might go against your desires, but I have seen way too many people wish they'd waited as they backslide or go through their own journey and then feel embarrassed as a result. Far better to introduce it to them from a place of strength and solidity than wobbliness and naivety for sure! In the meantime, there is nothing at all to stop you from *quietly* introducing more raw foods to your family's diet. The best ways to do this is via juices, smoothies, sweet treats and more salads. You can just say, if asked, that you want you all to be healthier.

There's one exception to the secrecy rule and that's if your partner is open-minded and you think they'd be happy to learn alongside you. If that's the case, great, it's not an issue and you're bound to have a lot of fun learning and experimenting together, but if they are the kind of person to be sceptical or less than supportive, then it will be best for you to go about your business as privately as you can and broach the conversation if and when you feel the time is right.

CATERING AT HOME

One of the best tips I can possibly give you about eating at home with others is to make as many mealtimes "buffet-style" as possible. This goes for regular mealtimes as well as when entertaining and will ensure that you get what you want each and every time.

In this day and age where there are so many different eating habits and sensitivities among us, it's not at all unusual now to have more than a couple of people at a gathering have special dietary requirements.

For this reason as well as your own, it's brilliant (and considerate) to be able to offer a variety of foods at the table so that there's something for everyone, and those that can eat everything do, and those who have to be more selective or choose to be are also more than happy.

The other great thing about a buffet is that unlike a sit-down dinner where everyone usually has the same meal, no-one is going to be ogling your plate and talking about what you've got because everyone's plate will be different.

This one tip alone will make for an easier life, I promise.

Bonus Tips
Talking of tips, here are four bonus starter-tips to help you make your dining experiences as enjoyable as ever and exactly what you want them to be from day one.

- Always carry a few extra raw treats or handy-to-haves in your bag, desk drawer or car.
- Keep a small box or bag of goodies to hand in your kitchen that you can just grab-and-go when you know you're going to be eating out that day.
- Know exactly where you stand with social eating: some people decide that this will be the time where "anything goes" so eating raw is not even an issue; others choose to eat some cooked food while they might not at home, and others keep it as raw out-and-about as they do normally. Whatever you

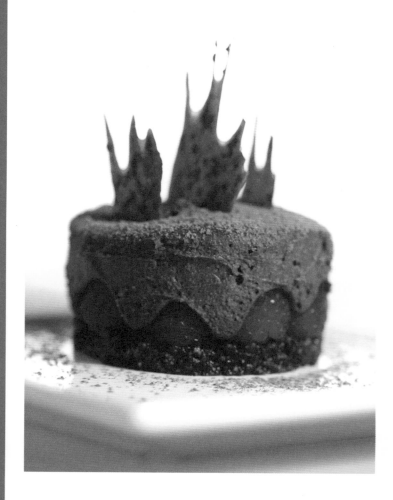

decide, make the choice that makes you feel happiest and prepare accordingly!

✪ Have a couple of "wow" dishes that you're really good at making and that everyone loves (and don't even guess are raw). A filling main meal like raw pizza is always a great choice, and a stunning dessert (like the one pictured opposite) cannot fail to impress.

A FINAL WORD ABOUT SOCIAL EATING RAW-STYLE

Most importantly of all, remember that every time you eat raw in front of someone else, whether it be one person or a group, you are giving others the opportunity to learn about something wonderful.

If you use the tips I have shared with you in this chapter, you will find that you can love eating raw as much in public as you do in private, and no doubt you'll have some pretty interesting conversations along the way.

Bon appétit!

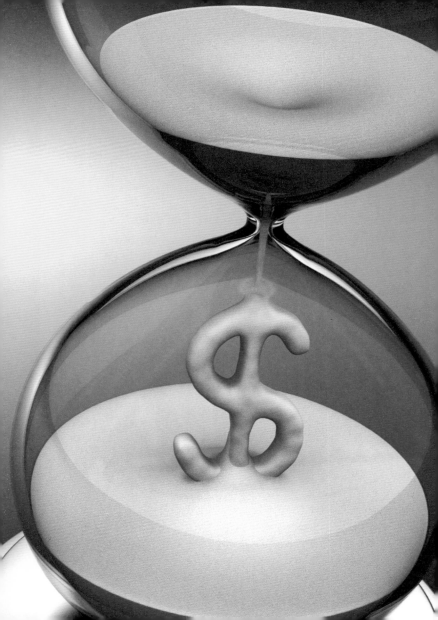

chapter 10
Time, money & energy issues

When people start considering changing their diet, not just to more raw foods specifically, but in any new direction, it's inevitable that the issues of time, money and energy will soon crop up as areas to be addressed.

As a busy woman myself, I fully understand that all three areas are those that just about everyone needs to pay close attention to. Indeed, the majority of people are time-poor these days, finances are also a concern for most and energy certainly is an issue for some 85%+ of the western world. What follows now are the most common questions I've been asked in each of those areas. Chances are they're the same questions that you'll be asking too.

"Will eating raw take more time?"

Not if you don't want it to. Just as you can exist off of microwave meals and be done in 10 minutes or can home-cook from scratch and wait an hour or more for dinner, the same possibilities exist within the spectrum of raw food. For myself as I am not one for spending hours in the kitchen, I spend no more than 30 minutes per day *total* taking care of all my food prep needs – and that includes breakfast, lunch, dinner, snacks and even on occasion, desserts. Not bad at all, especially when you consider that I am eating so much healthier than I would be if I were creating any kind of cooked meal in the same time frame. At the opposite end of the spectrum, some raw dishes, the more gourmet ones specifically, can take up to an hour to pull together like any other starting-from-scratch home cooked dish. And some other forms of raw food prep like marinating, dehydrating and fermenting can actually take 24 hours or more to be ready to eat. I personally leave that to the chef-types who enjoy that kind of thing!

With this in mind, know two things: 1) First, YOU decide how much time you want to spend in the kitchen on raw food prep and then choose your recipes accordingly; 2) It will pay you massively to truly understand that every moment you spend in your kitchen preparing raw food is a huge investment in your health and that of your family, and that rather than taking years *off* your life with your eating habits, you could actually be gaining them.

This last point is a big one. It is not uncommon for people to not only look and feel better within a day or two of eating more raw, but also to gain a lot of time and energy. Typically most people find themselves going to bed two hours later than normal, or getting up two hours earlier because they no longer need to sleep as long as before owing to their new lifestyle. Pretty cool when you think about it. So you can not only save time and energy in the kitchen when you eat raw, but you can also *gain* an extra two hours in your day, every day – sometimes more. That's certainly one of the big bonuses I enjoy for myself with the kind of lifestyle I live. An extra 14 hours per week come in very handy as a business woman, girl about town and mother!

Finally, it definitely pays to be organised. Making big batches of things like Raw Muesli, Veggie-Nut Burgers, Truly Raw Coleslaw, Raw Mayonnaise, Raw Chocolate Sauce, Mushroom Pâté, Almond Hummous and freezing lots of ripe bananas ready for ice-cream will make things even more efficient and "good to go" for you.

In the next chapter you'll find an example of a 5 Day Raw Lifestyle Plan that you can follow quickly and easily with minimum fuss or inconvenience, no matter what your current lifestyle may be. As you read through it, I invite you to note from this example just how easy and straightforward things can be for you, and to know that overall not only could it be quicker than your current food prep routine, but also healthier, easier, cleaner and overall more enjoyable to eat AND it will make you look and feel better than you have done for a very long time.

"Will eating raw be more expensive?"

Similar to the time question, you get to decide the answer to this. For example, you could spend your money on all the latest superfoods, speciality foods, imported tropical fruits and gourmet raw treats, and for sure you could spend a pretty penny in no time whatsoever, but if you focused instead on keeping your shopping basket full of the more local, seasonal and simpler produce, I'd be surprised if you would see any difference in your food bill unless you've been living off the value range from your local supermarket – in which case, take a deep breath, spend the money and know that you will feel like a million dollars in a few days compared to how you feel today. Plus, that extra energy, vitality and joie de vivre that you gain in the next few days once experienced, you'll soon consider priceless.

When it comes to bagging raw food bargains, here are some great tips for obtaining the best quality produce at the lowest possible prices:

✪ **Pooling resources with others** is an excellent way to save time and money. You can bulk buy from wholefoods wholesalers, pool your knowledge, and also take it in turns to do the shopping or ordering. You'll also find that when you order with other people, you'll likely try new foods you might not have tried otherwise and discover some really lovely new ingredients or main meal staples. And then there's the added bonus of feeling part of a healthy eating community.

✪ **Grow as much of your own produce as possible.** If you don't have the space or time to get into gardening on any great scale, you can still grow plenty of sprouts and indoor greens which can save you a small fortune (one woman I know cut her food bill by a third by swapping meat for sprouts). Also, as you have already learned, sprouted beans, seeds and grains also supply some of the most live and potent nutrients you will ever find, and for next to nothing in many cases. Visit **www.TheRawFoodCoach.com** for further details about sprouting.

- ✪ **Dehydrate many of your fresh foods** which are past their best, but still edible, but which you're not planning on using before they deteriorate further. Instead you can dehydrate them in a number of ways (slices, chips, marinated then dehydrated, dehydrated then ground into sprinkles and seasonings etc.) and use them later.

- ✪ **Freeze any bananas** that are speckled but not yet black if you're not going to get through them before they turn. Take the skin off and put in the freezer – within a few hours you'll have the basic ingredient for a great raw ice-cream or frozen lolly. Do the same with other fresh fruit – most fruits translate excellently into ice-cream or sorbet at a later date.

- ✪ One of the very best tips for saving money on a regular basis is to **find out when your favourite shops mark down their produce**. Typically supermarkets have a day and/or time where they reduce prices on fresh goods by up to 90%, and you can find some real bargains. You just have to know when these days are and what times are best. The quickest way to find out? Just ask one of the checkout assistants!

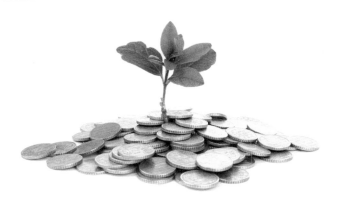

✪ **Consider advertising** or putting the word around that you're looking for organic fruits and vegetables that are locally grown. Lots of allotment growers have excess produce that often goes to waste - connect with them and offer to take the excess off their hands for pennies rather than pounds - top idea!

✪ **Choose to frequent farm shops** rather than supermarkets – many reasons why of course, but financially-speaking you can buy fresh produce that is twice as nutritious and half the price from local farm growers – and it's usually not dipped in chemicals like commercial organic produce.

✪ **Call a well-known raw food mail order supplier** and find out what foods, books and equipment are currently sitting in the "bargain box". Often these companies have nut butters and other foods close to their sell-by date that they sell for less than half price, or books that have been damaged in transit that cannot be sold as new.

✪ When it comes to buying books or equipment, **look out for decent second hand pieces** in the small ads section of your local paper, online, through e-bay, at car boot sales, or buy/sell via TheRawFoodDirectory.com.

✪ And finally, **don't forget the food for free options**, such as foraging for wild greens in clean parks and woodlands, mushroom, berry and apple picking, and so forth.

"How much energy will switching to more raw food take?"

First off, let's be clear that what makes any kind of diet transition laborious is thinking it's going to be that way. Not helpful! Conversely, if you go into it with the mindset that it's going to be really easy and fun, then guess what? It *will* be easy and

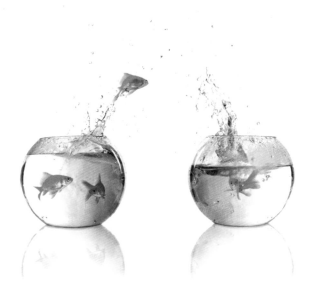

fun, *because you make it so*. Sounds obvious, I know, but it's amazing how many people get very worked up about changing the way they eat for a whole number of unfounded reasons and turn it in to a very big and complicated deal. The fact is, it *is* easy. You just need to know what to buy, what to do with it, and then… enjoy it! The fun part is vital for most people, it certainly is for me, and I think it's particularly important to focus on fun when upgrading your diet; otherwise, for many people it can become a very serious affair, and a lot of the joy that getting healthier can bring can be lost in the intense focus on "getting it right". The fact is there really isn't a "getting it right" because there is no perfect diet, only what works for you. And a big piece of that perfection for you is being in love with what you eat so you can feel great about it on all levels, not just intellectually. So I advise you to only buy foods that you love or think you might love if you tried it, and take it from there.

With all of the above said, it's hopefully easy to see why a lot of the "energy" that people use up when transitioning to a new way of eating is actually mental energy – and totally unnecessary. The stress, worry and anxiety that some people feel can be considerable. And it's a complete *waste* of energy. Why do it if you're going to get anxious about it? Just give it a try and put your energy into getting excited about trying new foods and new ways of doing things, and you'll find that you'll be *gaining* extra energy in no time at all and hopefully, having fun with your food and seeing as a grand adventure (which is what it truly is).

On the topic of *gaining* energy, I've already mentioned that you can easily gain an extra two hours in your day through eating a high or all-raw food diet. Not only that, but the *quality* of those two hours and all the hours preceding them is completely different. You'll find that you'll think more clearly, your focus will be better, your decision making will be faster and overall you'll simply get more done. No more dragging heels or huffing and puffing your way through your day. You'll be amazed at how the quality and quantity of your energy shifts, and honestly you will wonder how on earth you ever managed to get through life on the energy and mindset that you had before.

Prepare to be amazed!

So there you have it. Time, money and energy. The bottom line is: YOU decide. Get clear on how much time you want it to take, how much money you are happy to spend and get yourself in a positive mindset about your colourful adventure ahead and before long you'll be experiencing more of everything – and all it will have cost you is a change of focus and learning a few new things that will improve your life forever.

I think that's a trade worth making, don't you?

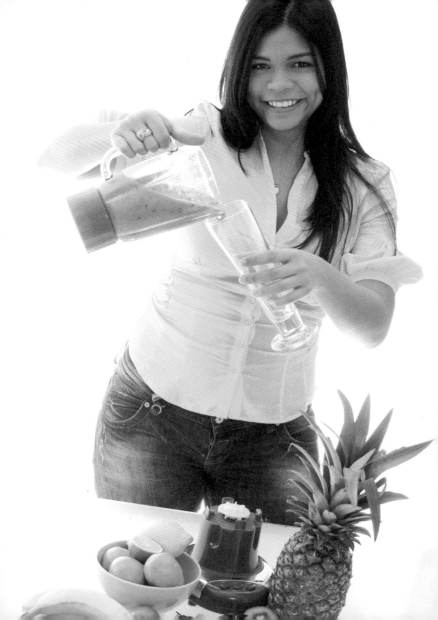

chapter 11
Your 5 day raw lifestyle plan

If you're ready to see and feel the difference that running on raw power brings, then here's the part you've been waiting for!

In this chapter you'll find a very simple 5 day raw lifestyle plan that will show you how to eat a diet that is three-quarters raw. I've chosen 75% because it will stretch you and allow you to experience some wonderful raw-related benefits, but will still enable you to eat some healthy cooked foods as well. Of course, if you want to aim for a higher percentage or even 100% raw, then simply omit the cooked foods I've listed and replace them with more raw foods or recipes of your choice.

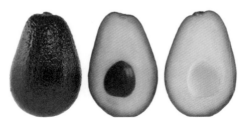

Before you get started, just a few quick pointers:

⭐ Choose a time to follow this plan when you have an easy schedule in front of you. If you try and do this while your life is especially chaotic, turbulent or demanding, what should feel fun will instead feel stressful and overwhelming, so pick a week when you have the time and space to appreciate and enjoy your adventure.

⭐ Spend the 1–3 days preceding the plan weaning yourself off some of the more unhealthy foods or drinks you may currently be consuming. This is not about going cold turkey or putting yourself on a detox, but you'll find it so much easier and more rewarding if you can go into it feeling clean and physically prepared.

⭐ Get your kitchen organised to support the plan. Aside from the obvious shopping trip to secure your supplies, this may simply be a case of moving your blender from out of the cupboard and onto your most regularly used counter top, or it might mean having a radical purge of your fridge or cupboards. Whatever it is, do what needs to be done and you'll be put in the right place mentally and practically for the five days ahead.

⭐ Consider doing this with a friend, colleague or family member. As you may know from previous experiences, it can make all the difference to share in a new venture with someone else. In this case you could share the food prep duties, go shopping together and discuss what's going on as it happens if you involve a friend or two.

⭐ Most importantly of all, remember to view this as an experiment or an adventure. This is *just five days* so you have nothing to lose and so much to gain. Step out with a smile on your face and an open mind to what comes next and simply let nature take its course...

On the next page you will find your 5 day menu plan followed by an explanation of how it all works together with the answers to the questions that you may have in relation to it. In Chapter 14 you'll find 15 quick, easy and delicious raw food recipes that you can use as part of this plan. If you'd like to print these out, you can find a larger version of both the menu plan and the recipes for download at **www.RawFoodBonuses.com**.

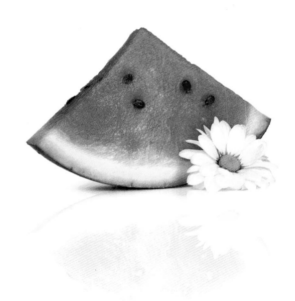

	Breakfast	**Lunch**
DAY 1	**Raw Muesli** served with homemade raw Almond Milk or shop-bought rice milk *(See recipe on page 130)*	Wholemeal sandwich, spread with hummous and filled with avocado, cucumber and tomato or salad of choice
DAY 2	**Mango and Spinach Smoothie** *(See recipe on page 132)*	1–2 **Veggie-Nut Burgers** with salad of choice *(See recipe on page 136)*
DAY 3	**Almond-Banana Milk** *(See recipe on page 133)*	1 **Stuffed Bell Pepper** with salad of choice or steamed veggies *(See recipe on page 137)*
DAY 4	**Orange and Banana Smoothie** *(See recipe on page 134)*	2–4 of **Karen's Favourite Nori Rolls** *(See recipe on page 138)*
DAY 5	**Unlimited Fresh Fruit** – whatever fruit/s you want and as much as you desire. Eat until full.	2 **Winter Cabbage Wraps with Garlic-Ginger Dipping Sauce** *(See recipe on page 140)*

Dinner	Snacks	Drinks
Choose any of the lunch options OR a healthy cooked food option *(See page 35)* with a salad/ steamed veggies	Fresh fruit	Pure water Freshly-made juices or smoothies (not pasteurised)
2–3 cups of cooked wholegrain rice with chopped salad and veggies of choice dressed with lemon juice and fresh herbs	Raw or super-healthy snack bar	Pure water Freshly-made juices or smoothies (not pasteurised)
Choose any of the lunch options OR a healthy cooked food option *(See page 35)* with a salad/ steamed veggies	Raw trail mix (shop-bought or home-made)	Pure water Freshly-made juices or smoothies (not pasteurised)
2–4 cups of cooked beans of choice mixed with chopped salad/veggies of choice. Dress as desired.	One small handful of nuts of choice	Pure water Freshly-made juices or smoothies (not pasteurised)
Choose any of the lunch options OR a healthy cooked food option *(See page 35)* with a salad/ steamed veggies	**Mango and Spinach Smoothie** *(See recipe on page 132)*	Pure water Freshly-made juices or smoothies (not pasteurised)

Your Menu Plan Explained

The recipes and meal ideas included in this plan are, as you can see, incredibly easy and doable and take into all the factors we spoke about in earlier chapters as well as a typical week's schedule.

As I have recommended simple everyday menu plans like these for years, I know from experience that if you're like most people, you're going to genuinely love this simple anyone-can-do-it approach. However, if there's something there that you just don't like or would prefer not to be there for whatever reason, then do feel free to adjust accordingly. This could mean eating or drinking something similar to what's suggested, swapping days or meals around, or leaving something out you don't like and replacing it with something you do. I *do not* want you eating or drinking anything that you don't love... otherwise what's the point? This is supposed to be easy, delicious and fun, remember?

As an additional focus, I also would like you to do your best to avoid eating when you're not hungry. This is so that you can really feel the benefits of the food. Overeating is never a good thing even on healthy foods. And while this is a challenge for most people, at the very least use your five days as an opportunity to see how much you use food as something other than fuel. Very enlightening!

By the way, don't be surprised if you end up eating less food than you thought you would. The more nutrient-dense your meals, the less your body will ask for as its nutritional needs are more quickly and easily met. (This is why many overweight people keep eating even when they've eaten a significant amount of food; the foods they have eaten contain "empty calories", and the body asks for more in a bid to be satisfied nutritionally.)

Let's now take a look at each meal of the day and I'll walk you through the suggestions I've made on the plan so that you can become more familiar with what's what and why it's there.

BREAKFAST

First of all, I don't want you to eat breakfast until you're actually hungry. That's rule number one! Breakfast is the most important meal of the day in that it's the one that sets you off on the right foot for the rest of the day – which is why your plan starts with a raw breakfast all five days.

On your 5 day plan I have given you many different breakfast options:

Raw Muesli

This is a very filling dish which will satiate even the biggest of appetites. If you have a sensitive digestive system or are not good with more difficult combinations, then you'll probably want to avoid this one. For most people it's perfectly delicious and satisfying. I've never known anyone not to love this breakfast; in fact many people eat it for supper.

Mango and Spinach Smoothie

Equipment required: Blender

Although these look very green, I have never met anyone who doesn't truly love (and feel much better for) a green smoothie. I'm sharing the recipe for my Mango and Spinach Smoothie because it's a firm client favourite and a true classic, but if you don't like one or both of those ingredients, then just choose a different green that you do like (even if it's lettuce) and another fruit of your choice. It's quite hard to get a green smoothie wrong.

Almond-Banana Milk

Equipment required: Blender

This is a lovely drink that you'll really enjoy. The bananas bring the sweet and creaminess to it, and the almonds make it more filling and fortifying. If you're trying to lose weight or have a nut allergy, no worries. You can easily forgo the almonds and simply make a thick banana milk – just as good only less filling.

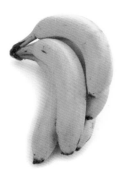

Orange and Banana Smoothie

Equipment required: Blender

So simple yet delicious, the orange juice and banana combination create a filling, creamy yet refreshing combination that is great at any time of year.

Unlimited Fresh Fruit

Unless you have candida or can't eat fruit for any other reason, then unlimited fresh fruit should work well for you. Do take professional advice if at all concerned that this might not be right for you. You can choose any fruits, eat more than one different type per meal, and eat as much as you wish. In fact, have some on standby as well, as depending on how new you are to this, you may be hungry an hour later! That's fine, just eat.

LUNCH

Sandwiches

I've given sandwiches as a lunch option because this is quite possibly the most commonly eaten lunch. That said, I've specified wholemeal bread (which I'd like you to adhere to) and to have a fresh salad filling. So this means no meat, cheese, pickles, mayo or whatever. My favourite filling is avocado, tomato and cucumber which is what I've recommended. If you can add in some salad leaves there as well, so much the better. You can have as many sandwiches as you want – use hummous as your spread if you need one – just keep it clean and wholesome! If you make your own, even better are wholemeal pitta breads as they are usually made from less ingredients and you eat less bread (and yeast). This is what I ate for months as I transitioned to more raw foods, and eventually I found that the bread started to taste much less appealing than the salad!

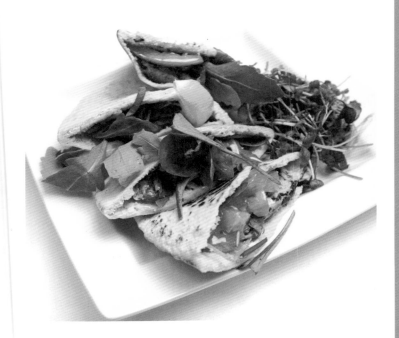

Veggie-Nut Burgers

Equipment required: Food Processor

These burgers are very quick and easy to make, extremely tasty because of the seasonings used and last for a few days in the fridge. These are a great option if you're looking for something savoury and filling to contrast against a salad and are a great evening option too.

Stuffed Bell Pepper

Another quick and easy recipe that has some stronger flavour because of the curry flavoured filling. Easy to assemble just about anywhere and easy to pack in a lunchbox, you can play with many different fillings as you become more adventurous in your raw food experiments and create even denser fillings from nuts or seeds if that's your preference.

Karen's Favourite Nori Rolls

These are one of my favourite lunches of all time. Not only can they be whipped up at your desk in less time than it takes to go to the sandwich shop, but they are also highly nutritious and low-cost. Truly raw nori is usually only available from specialist shops, but the toasted one you'll find in most health food shops and even some supermarkets is still a brilliant source of nutrition and is perfectly fine to get you started.

Winter Cabbage Wraps with Garlic-Ginger Dipping Sauce

Another easy-to-assemble option where you can take the basic ingredients to work and assemble in the work's kitchen. Cabbage isn't usually regarded as the most yummy thing to eat raw, but this particular recipe proves that in the right combination it can be amazing. Particularly delicious when eaten during the cooler months when lettuce just doesn't have the same appeal... Pack your dipping sauce in an airtight container and you'll be good to go.

DINNER

The evening meal is probably the one where you usually "let it all hang out". This is likely to be because you've had a hard day at work or have been run off your feet being a parent, so you just want to relax with a nice hot meal, something comforting and perhaps a glass of wine. I completely understand. We've all been there, and heavy foods and alcohol can help slow us down and numb us out quicker than just about anything.

During these five days, however, I would like you to do your very best to follow the plan to the letter and see how it feels *not* to drug yourself out or quash any remaining energy. Fret not, cooked food *is* still in the mix and you'll notice that I give you two nights with suggested menus comprising of a cooked carbohydrate with salad items, and on the other three nights a choice between any of the lunch options or a healthy cooked food option with salad or steamed veggies. When it comes to selecting this healthy cooked food option, please choose a food from those foods listed on page 35.

SNACKS

Snacking is not compulsory! Only eat when you're hungry, remember? That said, if you are not used to eating such "clean burning" foods as I recommend, then you may find yourself feeling hungrier sooner – this is normal, the body takes time to adjust. In this case, do snack. The snacks that I have listed are all super-healthy and will do the job, and I'm sure there'll be something in there that you love. NB: If you have a sweet tooth, please resist the urge to munch away on handfuls of dried fruit. These are very high in sugar, albeit natural, and can cause gas, bloating, and leave you feeling very stimulated; so go easy or avoid completely.

DRINKS

Often overlooked, drinks can do as much damage as unhealthy food. That cappuccino that is marketed so well can undo a lot of good work, as can that large pot of tea, the can of coke or glass of red wine, or whatever your tipple may be. For this reason I'm keeping it fresh, delicious and clean in the plan by recommending only pure water or freshly made juices or smoothies. If that's a struggle for you at this point in your life, then do your best. Even 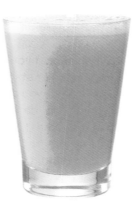 buying pasteurised juices or smoothies (99% of shop-bought ones are pasteurised so are not ideal) will be a step-up compared to what you might be used to drinking; it's all relative.

YOUR QUESTIONS ANSWERED

Now that you have your plan, do you now see how simple, easy and delicious eating raw and living food can be?

Even if you have the busiest schedule, YOU CAN DO THIS! Believe me, if I can do it with the number of plates I spin, then anyone can.

Looking at the menu, can you see any immediate problems? If you do, don't worry. Here are the answers to some of the questions you might be asking:

Q When should I do my shopping for this? Should I do it all at once or stagger it?

A Ideally you would shop every three or four days, but as this is a five day plan, you can get away with doing just one shop the day before you start.

Q I have candida and so do want to avoid the fruit. What else can I eat, and what can I use as a sweetener instead?

A Instead of eating fruit for breakfast or any recipe containing it, you can make a nut or seed milk by blending your nut or seed of choice with pure water and, if you feel you want or need it, adding a low GI sweetener that you know from experience works well for you. A green juice or pure vegetable juice is also a brilliant alternative, although less filling, so you could always blend in an avocado. You will either need access to a juice bar on a daily basis for this, or to own a juicer and make your own.

Q I am not a huge fan of green stuff. Do I have to eat it or drink it?

A Very rare is the person who loves eating lots of greens, but those who do benefit from it enormously. Green is the colour of balance, peace and healing. Think how much green is in nature, for example. It's everywhere and immediately has a calming effect on us just by seeing it or being in it. What is the middle colour in a rainbow? What do cows chew on all day that makes them passive and content? Green is the answer to a lot of modern day health issues, and the more of it we eat the better we feel, it's as simple as that. So if you are not a big fan of greens right now, do persevere. I didn't even like normal vegetables when I first started trying to eat healthily, and the only green food I liked was lettuce, and that wasn't with a passion either.

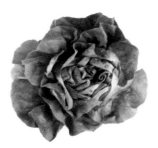

But over time as I got cleaner and my body and taste-buds rejuvenated, I actually came to crave greens and now love them completely. Some even taste sweet to me now; it's incredible. The green smoothie I recommend tastes fantastic, I promise you. You won't even know you are eating green (especially if you close your eyes!). Also consider taking a green superfood, even if it's in capsules so you don't see or taste it.

You can certainly stay alive without greens, but as for being truly healthy, you definitely need them in one way, shape or form.

Q I am cooking for more than just me. How can I adapt this meal plan to feed my partner and/or children?

A This is very easy. Typically you will probably be sharing the main (evening) meal with them, so it's a case of you following the menu plan for yourself, and if you don't think they'd like what you're having, then cook them one other thing (as much as they want) and serve that alongside the salad or whatever you have prepared. If they're a dessert lover, that's fine too. They can still have dessert, as can you, but you can pull theirs out of the fridge or freezer and you can prepare your own in a couple of minutes and everyone's happy.

Q What should I do if I "cheat" or skip a day? Does it mean I have failed or need to start all over again?

A I want you to "make like a toddler" and pick yourself up, dust yourself down and just carry on as if nothing had happened. Having the right mindset is really important when this happens. It is not helpful (or true) to see "falling off the wagon" as a failure or "cheating"; it's really not. It's about learning where your weak spots are, what drives you to eat things you don't want to eat, and as a great saying goes, "it's all information". No-one, but no-one gets things right first time or has no hiccups when trying to eat healthy, it's simply not human! But in answer to the question, when it happens, resist the temptation to think, "Well, that's it then. I've blown it. I may as well just eat the whole packet..." or whatever. Just remove yourself from the scene, and go and do something that uplifts you and makes you feel better. Decide that the next thing you eat will be fresh and raw, and follow through, and you'll be back up and running again in no time. (NB: If you are really struggling to do this, then chances are there's an emotional cause that's standing in your way. If this is the case and you're going through a tough time of it, then either do the best you can or come back later when your life is a bit less turbulent).

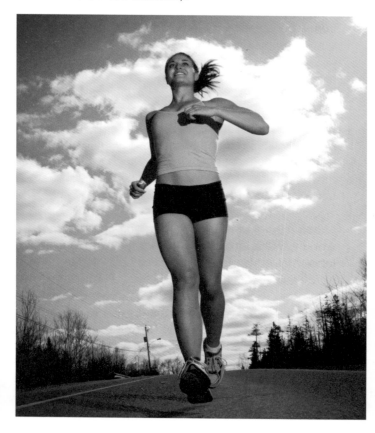

Q How should I be feeling at the end of the five days if I follow the plan?

A It all depends on where you're starting from and how closely you stick to the plan. If your health and/or energy has been poor to date, then you should definitely be feeling some difference by the end of the five days, but it may not be as marked as it would be in someone who is starting from a better place. It's important to understand that the body's first priority is to heal and stay alive. It usually won't give you too much extra energy to burn externally if it needs to put to use internally *first*, so you may need to be patient. That said, you may find that your energy comes in bursts and surprises you. I recommend that if you enjoy the plan and find it as easy as I think you will, that you follow the plan for a month and try to keep increasing the raw component as much as possible. Keep a diary from the very start so you can get an accurate picture – you'll be very glad you did.

Q I need a lot of calories owing to breastfeeding/ working out a lot/training/doing heavy manual labour. Will this plan work for me?

A Absolutely. Eat as much as you need, but be careful not to overeat. As you know, I only ever recommend that people eat when hungry and stop when they're full, but for most people this skill has to be relearned (we all had it as children). There is no limit to how MUCH you can eat of this food. If you need two pints of smoothie instead of one, then have your two pints. And come back for a third if necessary. You must never go hungry; that's completely counter-intuitive, which is what we're trying to align with here. So eat and drink as much as you feel you need and do not short change yourself – this is about learning to trust in the body's messages and then respecting them enough to honour those messages and give it what it wants. Some days you'll eat lots, others much less. Trust that your body knows what it is doing (it does) and enjoy the learning process as you ebb and flow with its requests. Yes, it might take a bit of getting used to, but it's a wonderful feeling to just let go and stop trying to control everything. Just go with it, and if you're worried about weight gain, please don't. Know that if you honour your hunger levels and don't overeat, you'll lose the weight you need to and stabilise at the weight that's right for you over time.

Q I don't like something on the menu and don't know what else to put in its place. What shall I do?

A You are welcome to swap any meals around or in and out. It's getting the variety across the five days that's important. If it's one particular ingredient that's the problem, find one similar to it in its food group that you DO like and use that. (Bag your free complete raw food shopping list at **www. RawFoodBonuses.com**.) If it's a general allergy issue and nothing from a certain food group is viable for you (such as nuts), then choose anything else that appeals that's of a similar ilk – in this case it would be something else fatty like avocado, seeds or olives. It really depends on what exactly you don't like and why, but of course you can always double up on a recipe that you *do* like and ignore the one that doesn't work for you completely.

Q If I want to eat more raw food than you've suggested, where's the best place to bring it in and what raw food should that ideally be?

A The order of priority would be:
1) Keep all breakfasts raw.
2) Add in more raw ingredients to your main meals, making one of them all-raw if desired.
3) Go all the way using recipes included in this book and on **www.TheRawFoodCoach.com** if you feel ready for a day, week or more on 100% raw.

Q I have a health condition and I don't know if this is a safe plan for me to follow. What do you think?

A As per the disclaimer at the start of this book, you always need to consult with a suitably qualified medical practitioner before embarking on something new like this. It is highly unlikely that you would experience any adverse health effects – in fact in most cases you would feel a whole lot better – but you need to err on the side of caution, so take advice and/or make changes under supervision depending on the severity of your condition.

Q I am on the road a lot and might not be able to make all the recipes as I won't have the food or equipment to hand. Any suggestions?

A I spend a good amount of time traveling internationally every year and can tell you it's entirely possible to eat raw or high raw just about anywhere with a little bit of forethought, planning or simply knowing how to think creatively on the spot. Many people travel with a hand blender or mini-blender. They're very small and light and

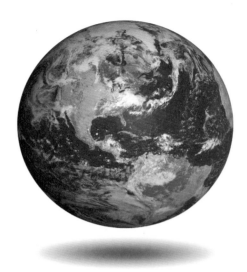

you can even get some that are battery powered, so you don't even need a plug point. These are very handy for all sorts of recipes and are super easy to clean. You can also prepare foods in advance, ones that will travel well, also stock up well on fruit, nuts, seeds, green powders, raw snack bars, anything dehydrated – anything that has some shelf life. There are ways and means with everything – you don't have to follow the recipes to the letter; just get the gist of them. The ingredients are what's important – just do your best to eat those foods somehow throughout the five days. Hopefully through answering these questions, I've made it clear just how flexible this plan can be. Remember, this is not a prescription, but a guide to get you started.

Q Can I live on the menu you prescribe long term or just for a few days? If so, would I need to supplement?

A Yes, this menu is absolutely viable long term as it is simply a healthier version of what most people eat already on a daily basis. The five days you have ahead of you is your opportunity to begin a whole new journey into foods and wellbeing that will probably be unlike any you have ever embarked on before. This first five days will teach you a lot about food and your relationship to it, and also how your body responds to different foods, but to really get an idea as to how this works and can benefit you, of course five days is but a drop in the ocean. If you choose to follow an all-raw vegan menu long term, then you may need to supplement. In fact, I would recommend you do, primarily because of the fact that our soils are deficient and food today is not like it was even as recently as a few decades ago. Most, if not all of us, are not receiving the nutrition that we ideally should. Going raw will improve matters immensely – and choosing organic where possible is important – but you still need to take care.

As a general rule of thumb, for anyone considering eating an all-raw vegan diet for a prolonged period of time, I recommend taking a vitamin B12 supplement and also a liquid vitamin D if you don't get a lot of sun. As always, take professional advice, and consider having some blood tests done early on into your journey so that you can see how your health profile changes over time as your diet improves.

The final thing I must stress is that it is actually possible to eat an unhealthy raw food diet. I have seen people thrive on raw food and I have also seen them fail to thrive. The latter group simply don't take enough care in what they eat, and think that as long as it's raw it's good or enough. That's not necessarily true. As mentioned throughout this book, it's vital to eat from a wide range of food groups and to eat the best quality food possible whenever possible. It's not enough to just think "raw". You have to think fresh, whole, ripe, live and organic too, or you will only yield mediocre results.

As time goes by and your experience and confidence increases, suddenly things that seem a bit mysterious now will all click into place and you'll have that big "aha" moment where you realise that this REALLY IS as easy as I said it was! Largely this is all just a case of un-learning some old patterns and habits and learning some new, more beneficial ways of doing things and putting them into action.

And talking of action, as we find ourselves now at the end of the 5 Day Raw Lifestyle Plan chapter, it's time to recap on everything we've covered and move into your *Go Raw! Action Steps Summary...*

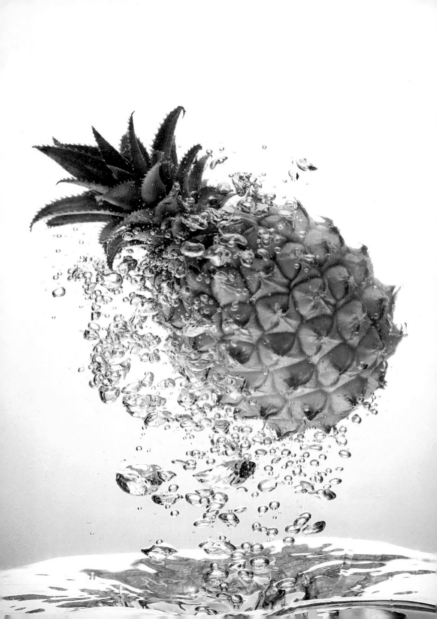

chapter 12
Go raw!
action steps summary

So, here we are – the grand finale!

Here's a recap of what we've covered so far:

- ❂ You've learned what raw food is and isn't.
- ❂ You've learned about the many benefits that eating more raw food can bring.
- ❂ You've learned that it doesn't have to be all or nothing, but generally speaking the more raw food you eat, the better you *will* look and feel.
- ❂ You've learned what a raw food diet can comprise of and all the different raw food groups that you can choose from.
- ❂ You've learned how to bring more raw foods into your diet in a way that is easy, simple and delicious, plus what are the healthiest cooked foods to eat.
- ❂ You've learned what kitchen equipment you should start with and why.
- ❂ You've learned how and where to shop for your raw foods.
- ❂ You've learned some raw nutrition facts, learned about the subtle and obvious benefits of eating raw food and what to be mindful of moving forward.

⊕ You've learned how to handle family and social situations in a way that works for everyone.

⊕ You've learned how to gain more time, money and energy through eating more raw foods.

⊕ You've learned what a five day raw lifestyle plan looks like and how easy it is to follow – and now you're all set to do it!

It's quite a journey we've been on together, isn't it? I hope you're feeling suitably inspired and ready to go!

If you're itching to get started, then this chapter will give you the ultimate checklist of things to do to get yourself set-up for success. Whether you choose to follow my plan or create one of your own, everything you need is here. It's just a case of joining the dots, doing what you love and in no time at all you'll be bagging those wonderful benefits and opening yourself up to a whole new world of possibilities.

Let's do it!

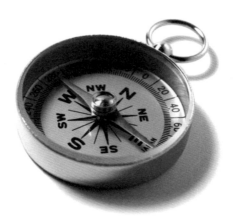

YOUR GO RAW! ACTION STEPS

✪ In a notebook or on your computer make a full and complete list of all the things about your body, diet and health that are currently bothering you, or are a serious problem, and that you want to be better. If you're really committed, also take photos of those things that are showing up visibly so you can watch them transform over the next few weeks. ☐

✪ List all the things that you would like to say are true for you in body, diet and health terms six months from now. How would you like to look and feel? How would you know that you were a different person? ☐

✪ Decide how much raw food you'd like to bring into your diet for the next week and write that figure down. (e.g. Half your diet, three-quarters, more, less…) ☐

✪ Download and print out all the goodies waiting for you at **www.RawFoodBonuses.com**. You will be needing these. ☐

✪ Using Chapter 5 as your starting point, make a list of five different breakfasts, lunches and dinners that you know you will love and that will support you in reaching your raw percentage and health goals. ☐

✪ Spend at least half a day detoxing your kitchen. The cleaner you make it the better you will feel instantly, and it will make it so much easier for you to make a fresh start with your diet. ☐

✪ Obtain the kitchen equipment that you need using Chapter 6 as a reminder of what's available and how to do this. ☐

✪ Create your own Rawganized Binder (see Chapter 6) and file any existing or new raw food resources in there so you are organised for success.

✪ Choose your favourite affirmation from the selection you obtained via **www.RawFoodBonuses.com** and pin it up in all the places in your home, office or elsewhere you know will make the difference. Make sure you keep one in your purse or wallet as well.

✪ Re-read Chapter 9 and decide how you will approach social situations moving forward considering what you know to be coming up and the amount of raw food you've chosen to eat.

✪ Get clear on how much time, money and energy you want to give to this project, using Chapter 10 as a reminder of what's realistic and possible.

✪ Re-read the 5 Day Raw Lifestyle Plan and decide whether you'd like to run with that menu, one of your own or a combination of the two. Whatever you decide, make sure your plan is on paper and you know exactly what you'll be doing when.

✪ Using Chapter 7 as inspiration, go shopping for the food and any kitchen items that you need to get started. Use the information in Chapter 8 as a reminder to go for the best quality you can find and afford, to go for lots of different colours, tastes, textures and food groups, and most of all to go for *life*!

Finally… It's time. There's nothing else left to do or say except those three little words you've been waiting for. Are you ready?

"Just do it!"

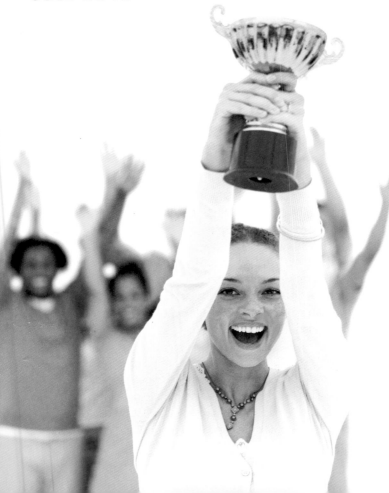

When you are complete, I recommend that you take a look back at where you were when you started and compare that to how you look and feel five days later. Depending on what you find, you may choose to continue for longer, up the amount of raw (or even lower it if the energy is getting too much!) or experiment with different recipes or ways of doing things that work better for your life and needs.

Remember, how much raw food you eat, when, why and what is for you to decide.

My only request is that you remember that at all times, and whatever you decide, that you do it with a smile on your face and are intent on loving your body and giving back to it as much as it has given you. Miracles are waiting for you when you start working with your body rather than against it.

Keep your mind on the positive and your journey will be a happy and healthy one – the feeling of taking charge of your destiny is amazing. In fact, the more you reflect on the changes you've made and the way that you feel, the more you'll be curious as to what's possible for you if you up the ante.

Are you ready to find out?

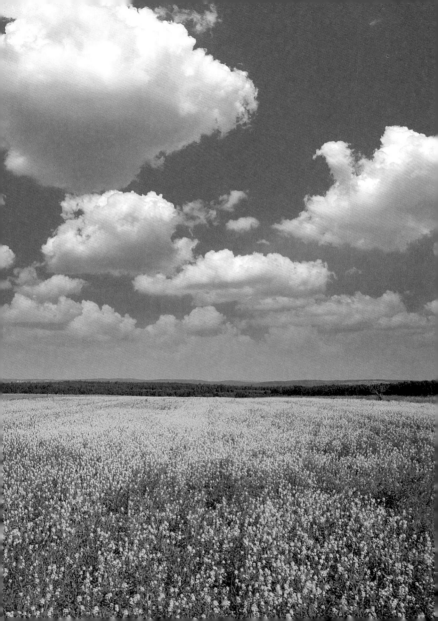

chapter 13
Final word: It's your story – you decide

Wow, we've come such a long way together!

We've looked at everything from the very basics of what raw food is, all the way through to how to bring it into your everyday life in easy, doable, healthy and delicious ways.

So, now it's over to you...

Are you feeling the raw buzz yet?

Remember, bringing any amount of raw food into your diet can only be a good thing, but the more you add, the more you will see and feel the difference.

From this point on you have all you need to transition to eating a high raw diet easily and enjoyably if you'd like to; beyond that is up to you.

BEYOND THE PLATE

So what *does* lay waiting on the other side?

Well, as alluded to earlier, once your body has had a chance to clean out whatever's been holding it back, it has more energy for other things. Fun things like... creating and living a brilliant life!

With your newfound clarity and zest for life, it naturally follows that you'll soon have the space, time and energy to look at pursuing new interests, passions and paths that will take you to even more exciting places.

Apart from the obvious health and energy benefits, it's this aspect of raw living that really makes it so worthwhile.

I know for me my whole life has changed because of eating more raw food. Not just in the obvious ways such as weight loss or looking and feeling better generally, but also in who it has helped me to become. The way I have come to see it is that you don't necessarily become a *different* person but instead a brighter, shinier version of your true self; you now have the energy to be more *fully* you, a more alive version, and to pursue those things you've always wanted to with a newfound courage and confidence that you can do whatever you set your mind to.

So, with a whole new world of possibilities at your feet, I do hope you will join me over at **www.TheRawFoodCoach.com** to learn more about what comes next, because it's a whole lot more than carrots and apples don't you know!

I look forward to meeting you there!

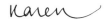

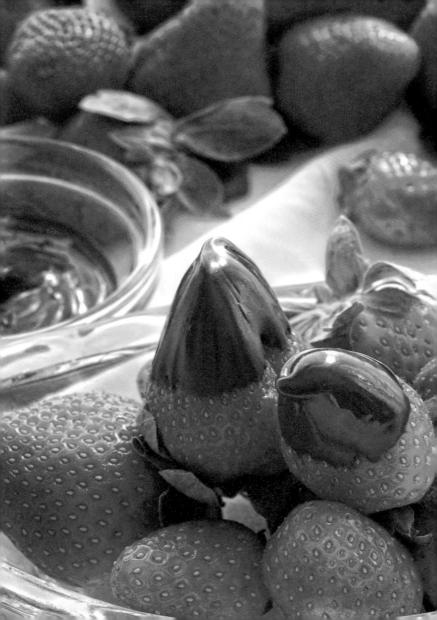

chapter 14
15 quick, easy & delicious raw food recipes

All of the following recipes are 100% raw *and* vegan and can be made with minimum or no equipment in 10 minutes or less – in fact, over half of them will take only five minutes.

You'll find most of these recipes featured in the 5 Day Raw Lifestyle Plan; the others are for you to add in as you desire or save for later.

I can personally guarantee that all of these recipes will be keepers. Quick, easy, healthy and delicious – all the boxes are ticked.

Don't forget you can download and print full-page versions of each recipe to put in your Rawganized Binder at **www.RawFoodBonuses.com**.

Happy prepping!

RAW MUESLI

This breakfast is one of my most simple yet popular recipes. Whether you are new to raw foods or simply want something really substantial that ticks all the boxes, this breakfast could really win awards. I recommend that you make a big batch up (minus the fresh fruit) and keep it in an airtight container so that you can dip in and out as you need.

★ Equipment
Blender

★ Ingredients
For Muesli:
1 banana, sliced into rings
1 apple, cubed
½ handful of Brazil nuts, sliced into small pieces
½ handful of hazel nuts, sliced into small pieces
1 handful of almonds, whole or sliced
1 handful of dates, fresh or dried, chopped into small pieces
1 handful of raisins (preferably pre-soaked, but not imperative)
1 handful of raspberries OR strawberries OR blueberries
1 handful of coconut chips
For Almond Milk:
1 cup of almonds
2 cups of pure water

★ Directions
1 Prepare all ingredients as above.
2 Place in bowl in the order listed above, saving some extra berries and coconut chips for later.
3 Mix all ingredients well.

4   Prepare almond milk by blending 2 cups of pure water with
    1 cup of raw almonds, then strain through sieve or nut milk
    bag.
5   Pour on milk.
6   Top with remainder of berries and coconut chips.
7   (Optional) sprinkle with any of the toppings suggested
    below.

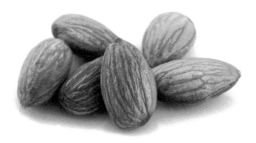

Some ideas for toppings:
Cinnamon; carob powder; mesquite powder; sprinkled raisins; nuts
which have been ground up in a nut mill; some raw coconut chips
or fresh coconut grated; a few dried cherries or goji berries or
other brightly coloured dried fruits.

Ingredients for raw muesli might be:
Apples, oranges, pineapple, banana, mango, papaya, peach, dates,
figs, prunes, raisins, sultanas, currants, coconut, almonds, hazel-
nuts, Brazil nuts, pumpkin seeds, sunflower seeds, sesame seeds.

MANGO AND SPINACH SMOOTHIE

Looking and feeling great has to start with leafy greens – it cleanses and rebuilds your body in miraculous ways. One or two glasses of this a day is going to make you look and feel amazing. And the good news is, it tastes truly – you're going to have to trust me on this! – delicious.

★ Equipment
Blender

★ Ingredients
1 large sweet and ripe mango or 2 small ones
5–6 large handfuls of organic spinach

★ Directions
1 Chop your peeled mango into pieces and put into a blender first (it's important that you put the mango in first as it creates the juice which the spinach can be blended into).
2 Wash your spinach thoroughly and add to the blender.
3 Blend the two together thoroughly until a thick but bit-free consistency is achieved.
4 Taste-test: If it's not sweet enough for you add 1–2 dates or more mango; if it's too sweet add more spinach.
5 Finally, if you prefer your smoothie runnier, simply add water to reach desired consistency.
6 When you're happy with taste and texture, pour into a tall glass and swoon! Feel the green goodness flooding into you!

I usually make 2 pints worth (the above recipe will make roughly this amount) and drink one immediately and put the other into another pint glass and keep in the fridge until later in the day. The latter makes for a great afternoon "snack" or a satiating predinner filler.

ALMOND-BANANA MILK

This recipe is delicious and filling, and very easy to make, especially if you use almond butter and save yourself having to strain the nuts first.

★ Equipment
Blender
Nut milk bag/fine sieve/strainer

★ Ingredients
1 cup of almonds OR 1 Tablespoon of raw almond butter
3 cups of pure water
1 large banana OR 2 small–medium bananas
2–4 Medjool dates (to your taste)

★ Directions
1 Place the almonds and water in a blender and blend until all the almonds are broken up.
2 If you use whole almonds and not almond butter (and therefore need to strain the milk) use a nut milk bag or very fine sieve to strain the mixture so that you separate the almond skin from the milk. When you've done this, pour the clean nut milk into your clean blender jug.
3 Add in your banana/s to the almond milk and blend until well combined.
4 Taste-test the milk. If it's not sweet enough, add some dates and blend again. Repeat until you find your perfect combination.

This drink is great for a breakfast, snack or light supper. This is best drunk right away, otherwise the banana will separate out and go slightly brown. The almond milk alone makes an excellent base for smoothies of all kinds.

ORANGE & BANANA SMOOTHIE

This recipe is about as easy as they come – all you need is a blender to make it and a hand-held citrus juicer is a bonus! Here's a really refreshing but filling smoothie that is bound to hit the spot for one breakfast time soon.

★ Equipment
Blender

★ Ingredients
2 medium bananas
2 juicy oranges (or 3 to 4 oranges if they're not so juicy)

★ Directions
1   Pop your peeled bananas into your blender then juice your oranges by hand and add in the juice.
2   Simply set your blender spinning until the mixture is lump-free and well combined and hey presto! You have one refreshingly different 2-ingredients-only smoothie. Yum!

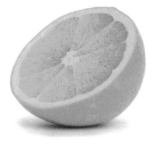

Use frozen bananas if you'd like an even creamier and cooler version. Double Yum!

FRESH FRUIT SALAD
with macadamia cream

A fresh fruit salad (done correctly) is one of the best meals on earth anyway, but when it's topped with this cream it's heaven on earth. Yes, really! The best Sunday breakfast EVER!

★ Equipment
Blender OR Hand blender

★ Ingredients for the Macadamia Cream
One handful of raw macadamia nuts
Juice of half an orange (or a whole one depending on juiciness)
2–4 large Medjool dates (or 4–8 smaller soaked ones)
Small piece of vanilla bean (optional)

★ Directions
1 Prepare your fruit salad using a wide range of fresh juicy fruits of your choice. A good mixture might be: Banana, orange, apple, strawberries, nectarines and blueberries.
2 Next, make your topping by blending all ingredients together until a thick creamy mixture is created.
3 Taste-test before using. Add more of whatever you need according to your tastes. You might want to add a pinch of healthy salt just to bring out the flavours a little more.
4 Serve your fruit salad and top with a good dose of the macadamia cream. I promise you'll love me forever for this!

This recipe will keep for about 2–3 days in the fridge. Great for topping some breakfasts for something a bit more sustaining, or why not throw a tablespoon or two in your fruit smoothie?

VEGGIE-NUT BURGERS

These are fresh and tasty "burgers" that require no cooking. Great as a main meal staple served with a large juicy salad or marinated vegetables.

★ Equipment

Blender (If you have a food processor or hand blender, even better)

★ Ingredients

1 cup of almonds

1 cup of pecans (use walnuts if you don't like pecans)

2–3 large carrots

½ large onion or more to taste

1 large handful of fresh parsley

¼ cup of lemon juice

1 teaspoon of Celtic sea salt OR Himalayan Crystal Salt
(or the healthiest salt you can find)

★ Directions

1 Put all ingredients into a food processor, or use a hand blender or table-top blender if you don't have one.

2 Taste-test – if you think it needs more spice, add some fresh or dried herbs or seasonings. Curry powder can work well!

3 Shape into burger shapes, either by hand, or using a mould.

You can turn this into a nut loaf by shaping into a loaf shape by hand or using a tin, or you can dehydrate the burgers a little or a lot to your desired consistency and/or taste. Crispy on the outside and moist on the inside works very well.

STUFFED BELL PEPPERS

Stuffed or filled veggies are a creative way to use some good fresh veg with something a little more dense, such as a nut or seed pâté, fresh guacamole or a nut cheese. These stuffed peppers make for a delicious main course and are very filling too.

★ Equipment
Blender

★ Ingredients

1 red bell pepper	1 avocado
½ clove garlic	1 teaspoon curry powder
Juice of ½ lemon	2 tomatoes

★ Directions

1   Slice your bell pepper in half and de-seed it. You may or many not wish to leave the stalks on. Alternatively, you may wish to cut the top off the pepper, creating a red pepper "bowl" and de-seed it that way. Both ways work!

2   Take your avocado and mash it in a bowl adding in the curry powder, lemon juice and crushed garlic. Give it a good mix.

3   Then, chop your tomatoes into small cubes and add to the avocado mixture.

4   Finally, spoon the mixture into your bell pepper and top with a sprinkling of any fresh raw seeds you have to hand such as sesame, pumpkin, sunflower or hemp. Yum!

Don't stop at bell peppers! You can use a number of different begins to fill in this way: Cucumbers de-seeded both ways, celery sticks, mushrooms, large "Beefsteak" tomatoes.

KAREN'S FAVOURITE NORI ROLLS

This nori roll recipe is a sure-fire winner and a recipe that I can live on for days on end. To find a recipe that suits you, use your favourite raw ingredients as fillings and continue to experiment with new textures and flavours. Makes 2 rolls.

★ Equipment
None

★ Ingredients
2 nori sheets
1 large avocado
2 fresh tomatoes
1 small onion
10 black olives, pitted OR 6 sundried tomatoes in oil
Handful of coriander (cilantro) OR rocket (arugula) OR
watercress OR sunflower greens (pictured)

★ Directions
1 Lay the nori sheet out flat on a plate or cutting board and place strips of avocado along the near edge about an inch in from the outside of the sheet.
2 Next, lay on top of the avocado some strips of tomato followed by strips of onion then topped with halved olives or the sundried tomatoes.
3 Finally top it all off with your chosen greens.
4 Roll up, either by hand or using a sushi mat, cut into small bit-sized pieces and enjoy!

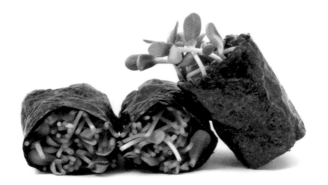

This recipe is just for starters. You can make infinite different nori roll fillings — just make sure that you have one "heavy" filling such as avocado, a paté or similar, and some wet and juicy ones like tomato, cucumber or bell pepper.

If making a nori roll that seems too full or has too many "wet" ingredients in it, use one large lettuce leaf to top the lot and then roll your nori — this protects the nori from becoming too wet and falling apart.

Raw nori is purple-black in colour and toasted is dark green. Truly raw nori needs to be purchased from a specialist raw food supplier. Don't worry if this isn't easy for you to find, just buy what you can — it's still really good for you and won't set you back.

WINTER CABBAGE WRAPS
with garlic-ginger dipping sauce

This recipe may not sound delicious (after all, white cabbage on its own is hardly a delicacy), but these wraps really are de-licious! Combined with the dip you have a really amazing combination, especially good for the winter months when you want more than lettuce.

★ Equipment
None

★ Ingredients

For the wraps:
White cabbage leaves
Avocado
Tomatoes
Black pitted olives
Coriander (cilantro)

For the dip:
Olive oil
Water
Lemon juice
Lime juice (optional)
Coriander (cilantro)
Garlic
Fresh ginger

★ Directions

To make the wraps:

1 Open the cabbage leaf and make a thick column of avocado slices down the middle, leaving a fair amount of space either side.

2 Pile on slices of fresh tomato, pieces of black pitted olives and top with a generous amount of fresh coriander.

To make the dip:

1 Pour a small amount (about 3 Tablespoons) of olive oil into a small bowl.
2 Add the juice of half a lemon, and, if you have one, the juice of a lime.
3 Add about 20 stalks of finely chopped fresh coriander, a small piece of ginger finely chopped, and half a bulb of garlic, finely chopped.
4 Add water to make the mixture less oily, but obviously do not water it down too much, or the taste will be spoiled.
5 Serve the dip in a tiny dipping bowl and your cabbage wraps laid open or secured with a cocktail stick. Prepare for true winter decadence.

Use this dip to give an oriental twist to the cabbage wraps.

Don't like avocado or don't want to use it? Nothing to stop you using a raw pâté or cheese in your wraps!

KALE & AVOCADO SALAD

This salad is an absolute classic. While kale may not be considered to be a great leafy green to eat raw, you'll be blown away by how delicious, filling and extremely nutritious this recipe is, not least because of the special method of preparation, which is super-easy to do.

★ **Equipment**

None

★ **Ingredients**

8 large handfuls of green curly kale

½ teaspoon of Celtic sea salt OR Himalayan Crystal Salt
(or the healthiest salt you can find that's not table salt)

1–2 Tablespoons of olive oil

1 ripe avocado

2 large tomatoes OR a handful of baby plum tomatoes

DRESSING: Squeeze of fresh lemon juice

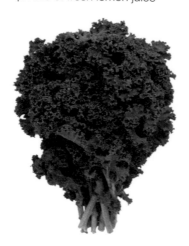

★ Directions

1 Chop the kale up into tiny pieces (roughly 1–2 cm square) and put into a bowl.

2 Add 1–2 Tablespoons of olive oil plus a small sprinkling of sea salt to the kale and massage well into the leaves until they are glistening and look succulent.

3 Chop up 1 avocado into small pieces, add to the kale and massage in well, coating the leaves. It is fine to leave pieces of avocado sitting amongst the leaves as well.

4 Chop tomatoes into small cubes and add to bowl. Feel free to add in any other raw ingredients that you may have to hand such as sliced onion, sundried tomatoes, olives or bell pepper.

5 Mix all ingredients well by hand – a very tactile and delicious experience! Make sure that all ingredients are spread evenly through out the bowl. Sprinkle with some fresh lemon juice and serve as is or pile high on to a plate and garnish with tomatoes.

By adding the oil and salt to the leaves the kale releases some of its moisture thereby making it much juicier in both taste and appearance. This treatment of kale makes it much more delicious and palatable, making all the difference for many people who ordinarily don't like kale as is.

KAREN'S FAVOURITE GUACAMOLE

Most people love guacamole, however it's made, and this one is guacamole with a twist. I've left out tomatoes (though you don't have to) and in comes the magical ingredient of cumin which makes it taste just divine! Mmmm. I could eat this for breakfast, lunch and dinner!

★ **Equipment**
   None

★ **Ingredients**
   2 ripe avocados
   1–2 teaspoons of cumin powder (to your taste, and depends on size of avocados)
   Juice of 1–2 lemons (depending on sweetness and amount of juice)
   1 small onion (red onion works better)

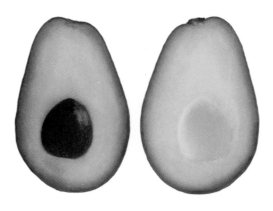

★ Directions

1. Slice your avocadoes in half and remove the pits. (NB: It's important that they're ripe – to check, they must "give" a little when squeezed). Remove the flesh and spoon into a bowl. Mash well with a fork, adding the lemon juice if it's hard going.

2. Add in the cumin powder (err on the side of caution first and add less than you think you might need). Then add the lemon juice and very finely chopped onion.

3. Mix all ingredients together by hand making sure the cumin and onion are spread evenly throughout the mixture.

4. Taste-test. Adapt as desired. If you like tomato in your guacamole, now's the time to add it.

5. When you're happy with your mixture, serve with crackers, as a side dish or as a filing for a wrap or roll. Yum yum.

Don't be afraid to add more ingredients to this recipe – tomato, red pepper, coriander (cilantro), basil, swap onion for garlic – it's all up to you.

If you're making a large batch and need to keep it fresh for a few hours, put the avocado stones (pits) in the bowl with the mixture and cover well. Refrigerate. All of these things will help it stay looking and tasting good.

FRUIT & NUT SURPRISES

It doesn't get much easier than this! These sweet treats make for a perfect, quick snack.

★ Equipment

None

★ Ingredients

4 Medjool dates (or as many as you want to make)
4–8 almonds OR Brazil nuts

★ Directions

1 Take your Medjool dates, cut or rip them in half, de-stone them and place one or two nuts between the two halves of each date.

2 That's it! The best bit is now to come...

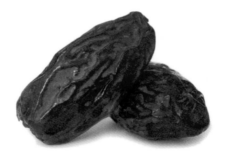

Try any nut in place of the almonds or Brazils. Great for snacks, after dinner treats, for children, for parties or for gifts.

CHOCOLATE DIPPING SAUCE

Oh-My-Goodness. That's really just about all I can say.

★ Equipment

Food processor

★ Ingredients

½ cup of raw chocolate powder

½ cup of agave nectar

½ cup of raw cashew butter OR raw almond butter

1 teaspoon of vanilla essence OR 1" of fresh vanilla bean

★ Directions

1 Simply place all ingredients into your food processor (this works better than a blender) and process into a thick runny chocolaty goo! It's a miracle! About 2 minutes worth of pouring and whizzing for the most amazing creation ever.

This is awesome as it is — just by the teaspoon (!) — but could be used as a dip for fresh strawberries or other decadent fruits, or as a drizzle for a fruit salad or raw cake or fruit pie.

Add a tablespoon to a smoothie or nut milk for instant choco-ness!

Add some raisins and/or nut pieces into the mixture for something a little more, um, "fruit 'n' nut"— like...

This mixture should keep well and happy in the fridge (covered) for a few days without any issues whatsoever. (If it lasts that long).

PS: Who needs a copy of "How to Win Friends and Influence People" anyway?

CHOCOLATE PUDDING

This is a super-quick and easy dessert that everyone seems to love. It's great for kids as the avocado is well hidden and can't be tasted and great for adults as it satisfies the sweet and chocolate tooth. Serves 1–2.

★ Equipment

Blender OR Hand Blender

★ Ingredients

2 avocados
½ cup of raw carob powder
1 cup of dates (Medjools ideally)

★ Directions

1 Simply blend all ingredients until the mixture is smooth and creamy and no lumps.

2 Taste-test before using. Add more avocado if you'd like it richer and/or creamier; add more dates for extra sweetness or add more carob for a stronger chocolate flavour.

3 Serve on its own or with raw ice-cream for the ultimate treat.

If you don't like carob then you can make this with cocoa powder or raw chocolate powder instead.

This recipe will keep for about 2–3 days in the fridge.

STRAWBERRY ICE-DREAM SMOOTHIE

For the kid in us all, this is a truly yummy drink that will satisfy any fast-food thick shake cravings or the yearning for something ice-creamy. Simple, easy and delicious (aren't they all?) this one is just divine. You just need to make sure you have your bananas frozen a few hours first…

★ Equipment
Blender OR Hand blender

★ Ingredients
1 cup of water
2 frozen bananas (peel before freezing and freeze until hard)
A small handful of fresh strawberries
OPTIONAL: Small piece of vanilla pod OR a few drops of vanilla
essence

★ Directions
1 Place all ingredients into a Vita-Mix or blender (NB: If not using a Vita-Mix, allow the frozen bananas to thaw for a while first, otherwise your blender may find it too tough to handle).
2 Blend all ingredients thoroughly until a thick whipped ice-cream like consistency is achieved.
3 Pour into a tall glass, serve with a strawberry on top, and savour slowly. Let the coolness transport you…

You can swap the strawberries for many other different fresh or frozen fruits, or use combinations to create your own special recipe. Mango and strawberry are lovely together. Makes for a lovely alternative to dessert — but always best eaten at least 2 hours after dinner for digestive reasons.

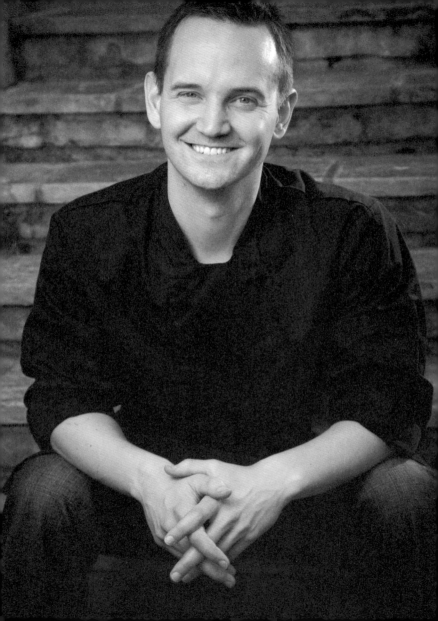

chapter 15
Raw transformation stories

On the following pages you will meet real people, just like you, who went raw for a whole host of different reasons.

Meet Ann who eradicated high cholesterol, high blood pressure, hay fever and more by going raw – and dropped 46 lbs in the process.

Meet Russell who went on a fast to clear up his skin, discovered raw food en route and went on become one of the world's most talented raw food chefs.

Meet Chili who lost over 100 lbs on raw and eradicated severe allergies along the way.

Meet Alejandro who transformed the health of her whole family through going raw for the sake of her daughter.

Meet Max who not only recovered from Chronic Fatigue Syndrome and Epstein Barr via the raw food diet, but became an accomplished athlete out the other side.

Meet Claire who discovered by chance that raw food not only rekindled her passion for cooking, but also brought extra spice to her body, her life and her libido!

Meet Kristin who traded Irritable Bowel Syndrome and lack of va-va-voom for a renewed zest for life and a whole new world of possibilities on raw.

Meet Kim who battled with embarrassing and painful psoriasis for years, was told there was no cure and after going raw watched in amazement as her skin healed and regenerated from the inside out.

Meet Lisa who literally prayed to God for a solution to her agonising lupus, was given raw food as the answer, put it into action, and has been in remission ever since.

Meet Mike who set out to find the ultimate nutritional path and went on a voyage of raw food discovery that's completely changed his life.

Meet Stewart who used raw food to achieve peak performance both at work and at play with very impressive results.

ANN PECKHAM, UK

"I grew up at a time when milk, bread and potatoes formed the majority of the average person's diet. When I was 15 I became a vegetarian on a diet that was very short on vegetables and consisted mostly of tea and toast, pizza and chips (fries). I suffered every winter with such painful sinusitis that I was in agony, and every summer I had such bad hay fever that I would rub my eyes so much that I developed big red rings half way down my cheeks.

"As an adult I hoped that things would improve, that I would grow out

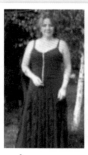
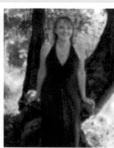

Before Raw   After Raw

of these childhood ills – instead I got rampant acne as well. Then I got acute constipation – so extreme that I ended up with an anal fissure which is one of the most painful conditions imaginable, and kidney stones which are also incredibly painful. To top this off I suffered from reoccurring bouts of depression and self-doubt.

"It didn't occur to me that all of my problems could be caused by my diet so I end up at the doctors being prescribed anti-depressants, steroid creams and anti-histamines – none of which worked. I was still depressed, spotty, overweight and dealing with hay fever.

"One day in 2006 I took the opportunity to have a complete medical examination. To my disbelief I discovered that not only was I spotty and in pain but I was nearly obese with raised blood pressure and high cholesterol. That made me so scared that I decided that I had got to do something before it was too late.

"I tried so many different diets to lose weight and feel better but I couldn't stick with any of them as they were just too restrictive and took too much time to work out. I was really feeling my age – I had aches and pains, shortness of breath and none of my clothes fitted me, so I knew I needed to try something new.

"I had come across the concept of raw food some 10 to 15 years previously when Leslie Kenton's book *Raw Energy* was published. At the time I had thought that it made complete sense, the notion that a living body thrives on living foods, but at that time there was very little support. This time around I discovered that there was a mass of information and resources and guidance.

"Since adopting a raw lifestyle I have discovered that there is so much variety in the foods I can eat now that I will have to live to be at least 200 years old just to try them all out. My weight has slowly but surely dropped off without any effort at all, so that I am now down from a UK size 18 to a size 10, losing a total of 46 lbs. along the way. My sinus problems and hay fever have disappeared since I cut dairy products from my life and my acne has almost completely cleared up. My cholesterol and blood pressure are now ideal and all without medication."

RUSSELL JAMES, UK

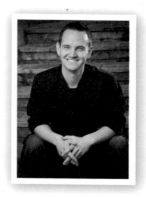

"I first came across raw foods in Koh Samui, Thailand, when I was on a seven day detox fast at a spa there. I can remember sitting in the beachside restaurant reading a raw food recipe book from their library and being amazed by the recipes in there.

"Now, it may have been the fact that I hadn't eaten for five days at this point, but I was fascinated. One recipe that particularly grabbed my attention was simply mango and avocado mixed together. It sounds strange but I was really blown away that you could do that with mangos and avocados! I read a description in that book of what raw food is and why it's beneficial and it made so much sense to me that I had one of those life-defining moments, an epiphany. From that moment on I was hooked. When I got home I went straight for the organic section at my local supermarket.

"Right away I started reading books on raw food and getting all the information I could. I actually started to get a bit overwhelmed and had to chill out a bit. It was at that time I was taking some serious abuse from people about how much weight I was losing and how stupid I was for spending all my money on organic food. This was from people that would spend double my weekly food bill on beer on a Saturday night out.

"But I knew I was doing the right thing; the whole reason I had gone to Koh Samui was to find a way of clearing up my skin from the spots that had started years before, when I worked in a fast food restaurant. I got that result very early on and could literally see my skin getting clearer each day when I fasted. That just continued to get better as I ate more raw food.

"The people I worked with at the time actually thought I had an eating disorder; they said that I was losing too much weight and in between mouthfuls of pizza and chips would tell me how they thought I wasn't getting all the nutrients my body needed. I found it incredible that they could be so concerned about me but not even think twice about what they were putting into their own mouths.

"Lunchtimes at work became 'question time with Russell'. I would get asked on a daily basis, 'What the hell have you got today?' That was when I was taking in a salad; you should have seen the circus that formed when I brought in the raw burgers!

"I knew I was onto something from the way I felt and looked so I just kept on doing it. I started eating my lunch outside, in the car by the harbour or anywhere that meant I could just eat in peace. That actually didn't help much because no-one ever saw me eat which made them think that I'd given up food completely! It's so funny now when I look back on it.

"I'm not around those people regularly any more but once they realised I wasn't going through a phase and wasn't going to 'change back' some of them actually started to accept it and even told me how they respected me for it. That was a great feeling.

"I continued to attend whatever raw food classes were available during this time whilst also teaching myself everything I could about raw food preparation. It was at this point that I had an email from Karen Knowler inviting me to work with her to create some 'raw goings-on' within her organisation at that time, The Fresh Network. That offer led to me moving to Cambridgeshire and being part of the hugely successful Fresh Network Raw Dinner Parties. From there I haven't looked back – traveling the world, training, leading and attending classes, meeting wonderful people, teaching everything I can about the lifestyle I love so much whilst always remaining a student.

"Today I am a full-time raw food chef doing what I love for a living. If someone had told me that this would be my destiny all those years back in Koh Samui I never would have believed them, but raw food has totally changed my life both personally and professionally, and I can't imagine living a life any more rewarding."

CHILI SCOTT, USA

"Three and a half years ago I changed my life. At 5'4" tall and weighing 230 lbs I was miserable and morbidly obese. I had life-threatening allergies to pineapple and cats which would stop my breathing and had to carry an EPI pen from my doctors with me at all times in case

Before Raw

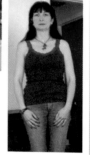

After Raw

I became exposed to either of those allergens. I also had hypoglycemia, and my blood sugar levels were never stable. Eating oranges or grapefruit caused massive blisters in and on my mouth that took weeks to heal. In a nutshell my system was totally toxic.

"Working as a fire medic and trained in medicine along with my Phd. I had more than enough education to know how dangerous and deadly allergies can be, as well as the dangers of the allergy medications that I was taking all the time. I had gone vegetarian and then vegan, but nothing worked to help me lose weight or correct the allergies.

"When I was introduced to a book about raw and living food, it not only changed, but saved my life. I started that same day on straight raw and living foods and juices. Five and a half months later I had lost 126 lbs and my blood sugar levels were wonderful and all my allergies were gone.

"I now eat pineapple daily and live with a furry feline friend. I also can and do drink orange juice and pink grapefruit juice as well as eat the whole fruits with no ill effects. My energy levels are way up and the way I felt when my teenage daughter saw me run for the first time in her life and exclaimed 'Mommy you ran!' was awesome! I now have the stamina to do so much more with my family and friends. I need less sleep and have not been sick in over three years.

"I have never had to count calories or fat or carbohydrate grams. I just eat raw and living delicious meals and snacks and love the new healthy me. This changed my life so profoundly that I am now a raw and living food personal coach, chef and educator teaching classes all over the United States as well as well overseeing two raw food restaurants in my spare time. I love the entire life change this has been for me, not to just lose weight and keep it off without the troubles and pitfalls of a traditional diet, but the change in my mind body and spirit has been so great that it affects everything I do and everyone I come in contact with. I am so honoured to show others the path that truly saved my life."

ALEJANDRA HERNANDO, MEXICO

"Five years ago, I didn't know anything about raw food, but my daughter knew better. She was born with many food allergies. She was breastfed but when she was just one month old she couldn't sleep, she was very colicky and

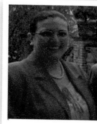 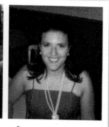

Before Raw   After Raw

she had what the doctors called "reflux". I got in contact with La Leche League in Mexico and was told that my baby could have a sensitivity to the cow's milk that I was consuming. I started my journey to raw food even though at that time I didn't even know it.

"On their advice I eliminated dairy products from my diet and my daughter started to sleep better and even stopped throwing up. We couldn't believe it but within two weeks she was another baby – and yet something was still getting her stomach upset so I began a food diary to see what made her sick. We discovered through this that she is allergic to cow's milk, sugar, soy, eggs, meat, fish, poultry, wheat, food colourings and food additives, chemical pesticides and fertilizers. Some of them cause an anaphylactic shock so we decided that we were not going to have that food at home at all and ended up eating a lot healthier.

"When I understood my daughter's way of eating, I realized that everything she couldn't eat we were not supposed to eat so we made a commitment at home about what we were going to consume and found out we were healing ourselves while doing that.

"My daughter liked to eat uncooked pea shoots before I put them in the pot when I was preparing a stew. She liked everything when I was preparing it, so when the soup was ready, she wasn't hungry. I just didn't realise she was eating raw food until someone asked if the girl was going to eat at the table, and I answered, 'No, she ate while I was preparing the food'.

"That's when I started to read about raw food on the internet. I didn't know how long it would take me but I knew I needed to eat raw, I needed to experience it for myself and I did it. Now I have a raw vegan family. My husband, my daughter and myself now are giving testimony of this way of living. This lifestyle has changed us all and now it's the time to touch others the way I was touched. It's my turn to give back what has been given to me and this is what I am doing right now.

"A year ago I started a website in Spanish to help my daughter spread the word. We did a green smoothie demonstration in a school and it was a total hit. My daughter told me that she was so happy to see that other kids liked what she eats. She is five years old and thriving on raw food.

"My husband has not used his inhaler for his asthma in many months now and I forgot about migraines, dandruff, heartburn, feeling tired, pre-menstrual syndrome and obesity. I thought my life was okay before, now I know my life is SUPERB."

MAX TUCK, UK

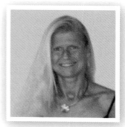

"My story begins in 1990 with a 27 year old vet who thought she was indestructible. Working between 10 and 16 hours a day, and always seeking recognition, this Type A started heading rapidly downhill, culminating in a double-whammy wake-up call of chronic fatigue and Epstein-Barr virus. My weight plummeted to 98 lbs and I had profound muscle wastage and no white blood cells. Immediate action was necessary!

"Having been written off by the medical profession, it was time to research. Fruit and veg was the answer that came to me; lots of it, and all raw. "Five a day" was for wimps. I was going to do TEN of each per day. I have no idea where this came from, only that as a child I hated cooked vegetables and would eat all of them raw or not at all.

"Twenty servings of fruit and veg a day didn't leave a lot of room for anything else, and my meat consumption fell dramatically. I had been dairy-free since age 15, fortunately, but food itself would not be enough to repair my wasted and exhausted body, so I started gym work to rebuild the lost muscle mass, and forced myself to go running.

"Initially I was only able to run to the next lamp post for fear of collapsing, but four months later I entered my first five mile road race. Feeling great after six months of a high-raw but not totally vegan diet, I went back to the doctor for a repeat blood test. The virus was gone. My immune system had recovered. I once again had a normal white cell count. My doctor was disinterested in my recovery and sadly five years later experienced a heart attack.

"In 1994, quite by accident, I stumbled across the concept of enzymes, which was a revelation. Further dietary changes ensued. I began sprouting. I ran marathons in less than four hours. I took up Triathlon, Quadrathlon, mountain bike racing and Karate. My body was lean and very strong. I felt amazing, and the need for sleep seemed to almost disappear.

"A few years later I read a magazine article about Karen Knowler and The Fresh Network, the organisation Karen was running, and joined immediately. I became totally immersed in the possibility of unlimited potential, and in 1998 became 100% raw vegan. In 2001 I climbed the highest mountain in South East Asia and gained my Black Belt in Karate, having fought, and beaten, an opponent 40 lbs heavier and considerably younger. Finally, in 2004, I fulfilled a promise that I had made to myself eight years earlier – I attended the Hippocrates Health Institute in Florida for their three week Life Change Program. In 2006 I qualified as a Hippocrates Health Educator, having experienced the most profound change of all – a deep emotional healing.

"I continue to educate myself and teach others in the living foods lifestyle via my company Optimised Living. I am passionate about living food and still feel that I have only just started to scratch the surface of my true potential. I would like to invite readers to my 100th birthday party (I am 47 at time of writing); it will be in Hawaii and we're going surfing!"

CLAIRE MAGUIRE, UK

"Going to the kitchen wondering what to make, yet again, was becoming a chore. It had got to the stage where it was just a merry-go round of never-ending food production for the family. I was, in effect, bored. This was a shame. I had always loved to cook. It has been one of my biggest passions. People loved my food. But now? Well, food uninspired me.

"One day a friend came to visit. She was a chef. We sat talking into the night about food – as you do! When she mentioned a green juice she had whilst in San Francisco, she said it was amazing, an elixir of life. Something in me stirred. It was an emotion deep within my stomach, and I knew that somehow this was the answer to my cooking dilemma.

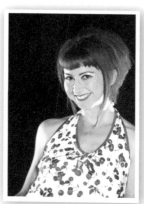

"Roll on a short period of time and I was on the internet. Surfing. What for, I really don't know now. I wish I could remember! But I found a site about raw food and it blew me away. This was it – my inspiration. I ran to the kitchen and looked at food in a completely different way. Boy, this was exciting. I created dishes upon dishes. Thai, Mexican, Indian, Traditional, Chinese… I re-invented all my favourite dishes in raw. Then I just plain invented new dishes. I found new ingredients; new foods that I had never heard of before. This drove me to create even more new dishes.

"My passion for food had been re-ignited. I was in love again… with making recipes!

"And then…

"The strangest of things started to happen. I began to feel really good. Not just a little bit but a big whack between the eyes, out-of-this-world amazing. And this raw food released me, because at that time in my life, mentally I was in a very bad place. I began to trust my inner voice, my guidance. I sat up and listened. And I acted. I grabbed opportunities. I shed my old skin and glistened with a new found beauty and confidence. I became hot on raw. I felt a sensuality and sassiness that was euphoric. Wow! I loved this raw food.

"And so my dreams slowly and steadily began to unfold. I trained to become a raw food coach as I was compelled to teach others the power raw food can have. Fun!

"And then… tragedy struck. A diagnosis of breast cancer. It left me shocked, betrayed by the wonder of life and my love affair with raw food ended. As I underwent treatment my body could not cope with the energetic force of raw. But this is no sad story, because as I emerged from treatment my body compelled me to eat raw food again. And so another re-invention occurred. As I rose up from the ashes my body responded to the playfulness and decadence of raw food. It stirred the femininity within me. I came face to face with the woman I had always dreamed of being and started to live as her. Hot on raw again. My message? That raw food connects you deeply and profoundly to your sexuality, so you can live, as I like to call it, as your Raw Bombshell. Are you ready to meet her?"

KRISTIN DOMIN, UK

"Two years ago in 2008 I suffered from many niggling health problems, such as irritable bowel syndrome (IBS), chronic fatigue, skin problems, no enthusiasm for life and I had not had a period in over a year – I felt like my body was shutting down. After many trips to my doctor, all my tests came back clear and I was ready to give up the hope of finding the vibrant health I wanted to achieve.

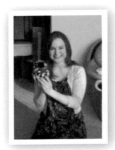

"I started to search the internet for

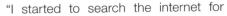

alternative routes to help relieve my symptoms but nothing had the lasting effect I had hoped for. I was introduced to the College of Natural Nutrition through a family friend and this was where my life really started to turn around. I changed my diet, cutting out dairy, wheat and sugar along with introducing various supplements and techniques such as castor oil packing. I felt like someone had handed my life back to me on a plate. My energy levels increased, my zest for life returned, my skin glowed and my periods were back!

"Just when I thought my health couldn't get any better I came across an article written by a "raw fooder" about her raw food diet – I was speechless when I read what she ate in a day (I thought my diet was fairly healthy!). Straight away, I went online and checked out her website which was filled with yummy treats and best of all they were dairy and gluten free – they even sold chocolate. I couldn't believe it, food that I could eat which seemed "naughty" but was actually good for you. I went onto every raw food website I could find and bought several books – I just knew this was right for me.

"I discovered raw food in April 2009; I am now one year on and the results are incredible. I rarely get IBS flare ups, I am constantly happy and energised, I love my life and I have learned to really appreciate the people that I share it with. Raw food opens up a whole new world which might sound a little crazy but by eating this high vibration food – your life becomes high! I am not the same person I was two years ago, I feel light, vibrant and alive. I have so many interests and have many goals I wish to achieve. It is not a diet, it is a way of living – I never ever count calories and the best bit? I adore what I eat! I am truly grateful to learning about raw foods and hope that by reading this, you will be inspired to start your own journey of magic!"

KIM RAYNER, UK

"I was diagnosed with psoriasis, a skin complaint, at the age of twenty-one. The doctor then promptly told me that it was a chronic condition that had no cure! However over the years as it worsened and became sore, unsightly, and open or infected I looked at alternatives to try and find a cure. So apart from standard steroid, vitamin D ointment 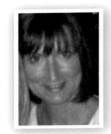 and coal tar products I also tried homeopathy, Chinese herbal medicine and daily U.V. treatment at the hospital. Sadly none of these things offered anything but a very short term slight reprieve.

"As I matured I became a mother, and even with changing hormones and work patterns the psoriasis didn't relinquish its grip. Then, during my third pregnancy I became a vegetarian for ethical reasons and was concerned about the effect this would have on my unborn child, so I asked my doctor if it was alright and she agreed that it would be fine but asked if my psoriasis had improved? After thinking about this for several seconds I had to admit that if anything my psoriasis had got worse. This I now know was due to my increased intake of wheat and dairy!

"Finally I stopped consulting doctors about it or using any medication and just learned to live with it as best I could and dress so that very little showed. I was eventually forced to contact my doctor when the psoriasis on my scalp was so thick I was afraid of losing my hair. At this point the doctor gave me a steroid solution that actually worked quite well – for a while – then it returned with a vengeance, so I asked my doctor for more of the solution.

"After using this bottle my scalp was open and weeping.

My just-washed hair would stick in clumps to the open wounds and would weep down my neck and behind my ears and I had to wipe at it constantly while I was at work. I was horrified and immediately booked another appointment and showed the doctor, who didn't seem at all surprised, and said that steroid preparations had this effect and to just stop using it. I was furious, it was much worse than it had ever been and I thought I should have been warned that this might happen. I decided at that moment to never seek treatment for this complaint again from a medical doctor!

"I went through that winter and caught four nasty colds in three months and felt very low and my psoriasis was always worse at this time of year. I decided that it wasn't normal to have this many colds and that I should take it as a wake-up call and look at my health myself. I began looking on the internet for anything to do with wellness, diet and detoxification and came across an experiment using raw foods to help people with a variety of medical conditions of which it seemed to help all of their symptoms. Intrigued, I thankfully continued my research.

"I discovered Karen Knowler's website and David Wolfe's book and gradually learned what a more natural diet should consist of and started eating 100% raw fruits and vegetables. The results were pretty much immediate! I had a week of low energy and terrible headaches that sent me to bed very early and my psoriasis patches had begun to spread even wider, but at the centre of each patch new, clear skin was forming and I just knew instinctively that this was going to work and that the psoriasis would go. I was now 46 years old and finally responsible for my own health!

"The psoriasis did go. Over the next seven months my skin got better and better until you could no longer see any scaly skin. I did not catch any colds and people started to comment on how well I was looking. I turned my attention to other subjects like the products that I put onto my skin as well as into my body and my immediate environment such as the products I used to clean my house with and made changes in these areas. I went to a party with my 21 year old son and was introduced to lots of people and one couldn't believe I was his mum! She thought we were all the same aged friends! My weight dropped and stabilised to 130 lbs which I was thrilled about making me a UK dress size 10–12.

"Some time later, I went on a beautiful holiday and ate an array of food. Some of it was cooked, but it didn't seem to do any harm. When I got home I seemed to have one celebration after another eating a bit more cooked food until I was virtually eating as before. Sure enough my psoriasis came back - I was horrified but seemed unable to motivate myself to a raw food diet for several months.

"I knew what and how to do it but couldn't get myself started until January and I was going to celebrate my 50th birthday that August so I began my raw journey again, this time without any problems and reached my birthday feeling fit and well. To date I stay on mainly raw food but may have an occasional baked sweet potato or steamed asparagus. I continue to learn and include various healthy practices to use in my life and feel that at my age I am just beginning on a new adventurous journey."

LISA LAMENDOLA, USA

"Living with a chronic illness can be hell on earth, to say the least. Listening to doctors doesn't necessarily help and I've learned the hard way that western medicine will only help suppress your symptoms, not heal your body.

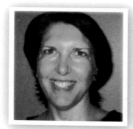

"My last lupus flare, over a year ago in 2008, was the worst I had ever experienced. Since being diagnosed in July of 2007 I tried every means imaginable to help my body find remission. The problem was, I wasn't helping it live past it. Then I hit the point of no return, and on a day I will never forget I got down on my arthritic knees and begged God for an answer, promising to tell everyone about it so they too could find answers. That afternoon raw foods entered my life and has never left. Through books, websites, blogs, and local health food stores I found a wealth of information, including recipes and foods I had never heard of, to lead me in the right direction – including a visit to the Hippocrates Health Institute in Florida. There I learned about my whole body, not just my intestinal track or immune system. I learned about life and what was missing from it and how I could get mine back!

"Changing the way I saw food wasn't easy, but each day I told myself to think about the alternative... not an option! Life is too short to just give up. After losing both parents to heart disease and diabetes I was not going to let my steady decline of health get the better of me. I was bound and determined to beat the odds. My Celiac Disease, Dermatitis Herpetiformis, Discoid Lupus and Systemic Lupus turned out to be a lethal combination against my immune system, putting me on the fast track to an early death. But by educating myself and diving head first into the raw food lifestyle I saw the most amazing healing take place. Raw foods gave me knowledge I never had before, about what food is and how it sustains the body. How sick my body had been all these years because it never got adequate nutrition.

"After two weeks of eating this way I was pain-free and after six weeks I didn't recognise the person looking back in the mirror! I looked amazing, my skin glowed, and as a bonus I lost 33 lbs! Sure I slacked off and started eating cooked foods again, especially in the winter, but when I started to feel sluggish I scared myself straight! So I immediately got back to the good foods!

"Now it is exactly one year to the day that I went into remission and I've never forgotten about my promise to God. I have made it my mission in life to help others find their own answers through my personal blog, *Lupus Girl Goes Raw* and now my new website and radio show. It is my hope to help others heal themselves and know how amazing life really is."

MIKE NASH, UK

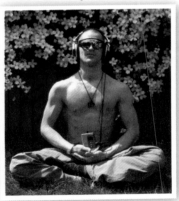

"From an early age I was fascinated by human behaviour and what separated those who appeared successful from those who appeared to be struggling. The concept of role models really made sense to me. If someone looked good, felt good and was achieving the results they wanted, then I wanted to know more. If someone talked a good game but didn't appear to be walking their talk, I tuned out quickly.

"I worked in the health industry from the age of 17 and

during this time developed and overwhelming passion for Neuro-Linguistic Programming (N.L.P.), hypnosis and mind technology. These approaches became useful in helping many of my clients achieve more of their health and fitness goals. As time went on I developed an addiction to helping people and began asking the question, 'How can I help more people?' The realisation was simple: To learn more. It was at this time I began studying nutrition in more depth. My hypothesis was that if a person combined exceptional nutrition with peak performance brain states they'd be able to do pretty much anything. I knew the power of energy, motivation, drive and desire, but I also knew that without adequate rest and relaxation, success could be short-lived and burn-out could become a very real possibility.

"My study of nutrition took many twists and turns. The one approach that captured my attention was the raw food diet. Every part of it made sense. The only problem I had was that I lost a huge amount of muscle mass on the diet and my recovery from exercise suffered. Looking back now I realise that at the time I was following a high-fruit raw diet. When I shifted the emphasis to more vegetables and greens I began to see a radical difference. This gave me a critical insight. It's not the just about 'the raw food diet', it's about how a person applies it that makes all the difference.

"During this time I was putting together my book *Aggressive Health* and began studying live blood analysis and more importantly bioterrain analysis. Bioterrain analysis had one simple premise: Unless the numbers of health were in place (electrolyte balance, anabolic/catabolic balance, pH levels, electron activity, energy balance etc.), it didn't matter what a person's religious beliefs were, or their spiritual tendencies, or what foods passed their lips; ultimately they would struggle with their health. It was a wake-up call that made me realise that even though the raw food approach appeared to be the most common sense, logical and ethical approach to the nutritional aspect of health, if someone didn't learn how to make it work for them, it could actually cause more problems than it resolved.

"During the last eight years since my book was released I've continued to develop my strength, health and knowledge of what works best for me. A typical day will include a regular green/vegetable based juice, a green based smoothie powered up with a variety of powerful green superfoods and a superfood-based smoothie. This isn't all I have in a single day, but represents my base-line standard. I'm not a raw-fooder and don't like 'labels'. I'm not a vegan and I'm not a vegetarian, although raw and living foods do form the majority of what I consume. Ultimately my approach is to help people 'Feel as good as they can as much as they can'. If someone is willing to experiment with all that is out there they'll find a way to make it work for them. If they are still struggling with their health, then they need to seek a practitioner who can help them investigate their biological terrain further. Sometimes one small tweak can make all the difference."

STEWART LYNCH, UK

"One of my first memories was at the age of five, when my parents asked me if I wanted to be vegetarian. I remember thinking it seemed like a good idea. They said that they had chosen to become vegetarian, and that although I would get vegetarian food at home I could eat whatever I liked when I was out. I always chose to stay vegetarian.

"My next change came when I met my girlfriend Max in

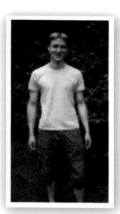

2000. Max was already raw, but I wasn't ready to try that straight away. However, at Max's recommendation I did become vegan, which immediately cleared up some minor skin problems. I then attended a seminar on raw food by David Wolfe, which was to change my life.

"I was so inspired that I decided to be 100% raw from that day. Initially I had decided to try it for one month. By the end of the month I had experienced so many benefits that I didn't want to return to cooked food.

"The first major benefit that I noticed was in my Karate training. I'd been doing Karate for 12 years. Within two weeks my flexibility had noticeably improved. The longer I stayed raw the more energy I had. Training up to five times a week, I was also working out at the gym, running, and climbing – my energy levels were through the roof.

"Probably the biggest benefit that I found was clarity of thought, which in my job as a computer programmer is a real benefit. My job at the time was potentially very stressful with long hours. I remember often working through the night, getting only two or three hours sleep, and walking into meetings the next morning still fresh and productive. This continued for weeks at a time. On one occasion I juice fasted for four days and was more productive than I'd ever been. Thankfully I have a much better work-life balance now, but it really opened my eyes as to what I could achieve on raw food.

"Other benefits that I have found over the years are: never getting ill, needing less sleep, increased stamina, improved recovery times, and enjoying my food. An unexpected benefit was becoming more in touch with nature, and having a more spiritual outlook on life.

"As with anything in life, the ripples spread out. My mum became raw and is now a raw food coach. My sister Catherine uses raw food to help her with her M.E. I also regularly help out with raw events and Max's talks and website. I am very fortunate to be surrounded by like-minded people and we all support and encourage each other.

"I'm currently stronger, fitter and healthier than I've ever been. I've been raw for 10 years and wouldn't ever consider going back to a standard diet. Most of the time I don't even think about raw, it's just what I do. Many people come to the raw diet because of an illness, but my approach is about taking health to another level. I have so many interests and activities now that there are not enough hours in the day. Raw food gives me the drive and energy to live life to the full."

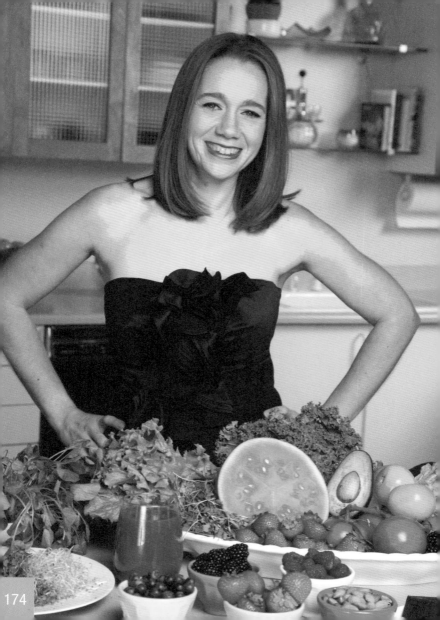

About the author

Karen Knowler is The Raw Food Coach, former Managing Director of The Fresh Network, the UK's original raw and living foods organisation, creator and former editor of *Get Fresh!* magazine and creator of TheRawFoodDirectory.com, the ultimate one-stop international online raw food directory. A raw food fan since she first discovered the concept of eating raw in 1993 aged 20, Karen has been teaching, writing and coaching professionally on raw foods since 1998. Owing to her groundbreaking work in the field of raw foods and human potential and dubbed "The world's premier raw food coach", Karen now trains others how to become world-class raw food coaches and teachers via her trainings and home study programs.

Author of **Raw Food Made Simple** and creator of numerous life-changing programs, articles and ePublications, Karen has lectured around the world, has been seen by over 6 million viewers live on national TV, appears frequently in the national press and has coached and worked with people from all backgrounds including well-known celebrities.

Karen's extensive knowledge and experience of all issues relating to raw food eating, as well as her accessible, positive and inspiring take on "eating for energy" make her one of the most sought-after raw and living foods educators in the world today.

Karen lives near Cambridge, England. Learn more about Karen at **www.KarenKnowler.com**.

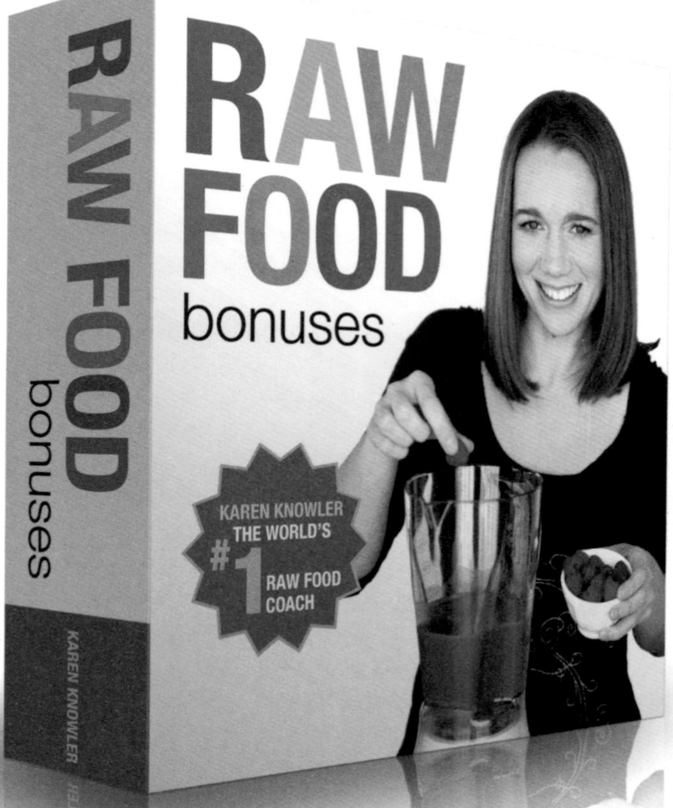
RAW FOOD
bonuses
KAREN KNOWLER
RAW
FOOD
bonuses
KAREN KNOWLER
THE WORLD'S
#1
RAW FOOD
COACH

Want more raw?

If you've enjoyed this book and want to learn more about how to go successfully raw, here's what you can do right away:

✪ Go to **www.RawFoodBonuses.com** to collect your free gift package of downloads including quick, easy and delicious raw food recipes, menu plans, posters and much more.

✪ Visit Karen's web site **www.TheRawFoodCoach.com** to learn more about how to go raw and bag some more great free stuff. (If you don't bag the freebies above then don't forget to sign-up for Karen's eZine "Successfully Raw" – you'll love the free articles and the quick and delicious recipes to add to your collection).

✪ Check out Karen's latest events, programs and products at **www.TheRawFoodCoach.com** – there'll be something that's a perfect fit for you and the next stage of your journey no matter what your budget or where you're at right now.

If you love this book...

If you've enjoyed this book and have found it valuable, chances are you may want to give some away as gifts to friends and loved ones – or in fact anyone else who bombards you with constant "so what about...?" questions.

This book was written especially to answer all those early questions, the ones we all ask at the beginning when we first hear about raw food and the raw food diet and specifically, how to get started. Well, now you don't need to be the one who has to come up with all the answers – let this little book do all the talking for you.

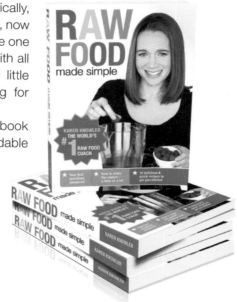

We've made this book both small and affordable so that turning other people on to raw food is easy and stress-free. Just hand them a copy and say "all your answers are right here – enjoy!"

They'll thank you for it later!

If you want to spread the word in other ways, here's how you can help:

- ⭐ Tell your local health food store about it and encourage them to stock it (print off a flyer at **www.RawFoodMadeSimpleBook.com** so they know what it's about and how to get it).
- ⭐ Tell your facebook and twitter friends about it – pull out a quote, share a tip or simply rave about it – we appreciate all of it.
- ⭐ Recommend it in your newsletter if you have one or to any chat groups or forums you may participate in.
- ⭐ If you'd like signed copies, you can order them via **www.TheRawFoodCoach.com** for the regular price plus shipping and handling.

WHOLESALE ENQUIRIES

To order copies in bulk simply order via Amazon as normal or for orders of 20 copies or more visit **www.RawFoodMadeSimpleBook.com** to get our special wholesale discounts.

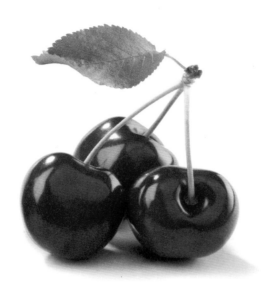

Thank you

Thank you to all at Pentacor for the design flair and attention that was brought to this book in painstaking detail. It is beautiful because of you!

Thank you to my friend and colleague Russell James for his fantastic raw food creations and the dessert photos he generously contributed, which are featured throughout this book.

Thank you to everyone who contributed their stories to Chapter 15, even those whose stories did not make it. You are ALL an inspiration!

And thank you to everyone who supported me in the writing of the book – friends, team, colleagues and more – having you behind me gave me what I needed to stay passionate at every stage. I hope you agree it was worth it.

Finally, thank YOU for taking the time to read this book and invest in your life and health this way. I hope I have the pleasure of meeting you or hearing from you one day.